Christianity & Bioethics

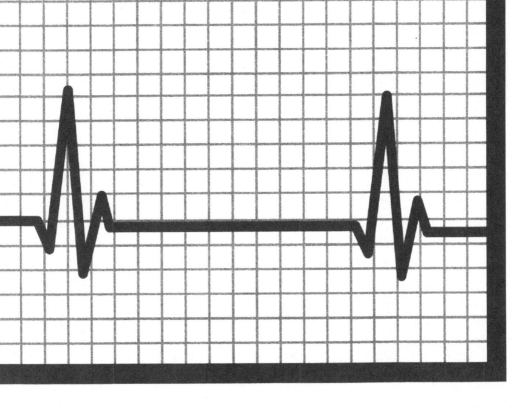

Christianity & Bioethics

Confronting Clinical Issues

Mark W. Foreman

College Press Publishing Company • Joplin, Missouri

Copyright © 1999
College Press Publishing Company
Reprint 2008

Printed and Bound in the United States of America
All Rights Reserved

Cover Design: Mark A. Cole

International Standard Book Number: 978-0-89900-755-7
The Library of Congress·has previously catalogued this book as follows:

Library of Congress Cataloging-in-Publication Data

Foreman, Mark W. (Mark Wesley), 1954–
   Christianity & bioethics: confronting clinical issues / Mark W.
Foreman.
     p.   cm.
   Includes bibliographical references.
   ISBN 0-89900-755-4 (paperback)
    1. Medical ethics—Religious aspects—Christianity. 2. Bioethics—
Religious aspects—Christianity. 3. Christian ethics. I. Title. II.
Title: Christianity and bioethics.
   R725.56.F67 1999
   174'.2—dc21
                                          99-24048
                                            CIP

To

Erin, Lindsay, and Kelly

who fill my life

with joy and meaning

TABLE OF CONTENTS

PREFACE

In an essay entitled, "Contemporary Christian Responsibility," Charles Colson throws down this challenge: "Christians must develop a well-reasoned Christian apologetic on all issues, and of course prominently the issues of bioethics."[1] This book is an attempt to take up that challenge. Because it is an apologetic, it aspires to offer a reasonable defense of a Christian perspective on certain issues in **bioethics**. However, its spirit is not one of confrontational dogmatism, but of concerned dialogue. It defends, but is not defensive.

One can barely read a newspaper or watch television these days without encountering controversial medical issues. Medical technology and new treatments are being discovered and promoted at a much faster rate than our ability to reflect on their ethical, social, legal and religious implications. As a result people are often unprepared to make the difficult choices that confront them today: Is abortion ever justifiable? If a loved one is suffering, can we take actions that might relieve their suffering but will hasten their death? Should doctors be allowed to help patients who wish to end their lives? If a child is severely impaired, can we allow it to die rather than face a life of suffering? Can we use genetic therapy to enhance the human race? Should we seriously consider **cloning** human beings? The way we answer these questions is indicative of who we are and what kind of world we want for ourselves and our children.

This book addresses these questions from a Christian perspective that is evangelical and conservative. I realize not everyone will agree with every point in it. For those who disagree with me, I welcome you. My hope is that you will consider my arguments and that this book will be a catalyst for further discussion and reflection into these issues.

I have written this book as an introduction into issues in bioethics. As such, it requires no prior knowledge on the part of the reader. I begin with a chapter introducing the basics of bioethics, ethical reasoning, and ethical theories. Each of the following chapters examines the legal and ethical implications of a specific issue in bioethics. I selected the particular topics covered in this book on the basis of their social significance; these seem to be the perennial issues in bioethical discussions. There are many other issues I could have included and perhaps will in a revised edition. For the time being, there is certainly enough here to mull over.

At the end of each chapter are references for further investigation. I have included a broad range of sources, and their inclusion should not be taken as an endorsement of their position. I have also included a number of websites. At the time of this writing, all these websites were accessible. However, as most computer-literate people are aware, the worldwide web is constantly in a state of flux and so there is no guarantee that these sites will always be available.

Terms which may be less familiar to the reader have been defined in a Glossary at the back of the book. These terms are printed in **boldface** in the text at their first occurrence.

Finally, this book would not have come about if it had not been for the help and support of a number of friends and colleagues. I first want to thank all my bioethics students with whom I have had fruitful discussions and who have given me the pleasure of having a part in their education. I also want to thank members of my department who continue to challenge me into refining my arguments. Specifically I want to express my deep appreciation to my mentors who have had a lasting impact on my thinking: Gary Habermas, J.P. Moreland, Norman Geisler, Francis J. Beckwith, and James Childress. I also want to thank two close friends who consistently exemplify

Christian love to me through their encouragement, support and downright tenacity, Wayne Pirmann and Harry Keith. Thanks also to John Hunter at College Press who stood behind me cracking the whip to keep me on track in finishing this project. Finally, a big thank you to Mark Carr, Janet Polarek, and my wife for reading through large sections of this manuscript and making many editorial corrections. Their help is sincerely appreciated.

Sola Deo Gloria
Mark W. Foreman
February, 1999

NOTES

[1]Charles W. Colson, "Contemporary Christian Responsibility," in *Genetic Ethics: Do the Ends Justify the Genes?* ed. by John F. Kilner, Rebecca D. Pentz, and Frank E. Young (Grand Rapids: Eerdmans, 1997), p. 226.

There is no end of good causes in the world,
and they would sorely tempt us
even if we did not live in a society
for which the pursuit of health has become a god,
justifying almost anything.

Gilbert Meilaender

CHAPTER 1

Modern Medicine in a Moral Fog

Modern Medicine in a Moral Fog

1

The 249 passengers of KLM Flight #4805 were waiting in eager anticipation to continue on to their final destination — Los Palmas Airport on Grand Canary Island. Los Palmas Airport had been closed due to a bomb threat and so the Dutch flight was diverted to the smaller Los Rodeos Airport on neighboring Tenerife Island, one of the string of Canary Islands that sat off the coast of Morocco. They waited for four hours until the Los Palmas airport was reopened. Now they were only 40 minutes from completing their flight.

As the 747 jumbo jet pulled from the gate, Captain Veldhuyzen Van Zanten peered through the thick fog that had just descended on the small airport that early March evening and lurched the plane full of vacationing passengers down the runway to taxi into place. Because of the closing of the main airport, this smaller airport was so overcrowded that planes had to taxi on the runway rather than the taxiway. Also on the runway that morning was Pan Am Flight #1736. Among its 394 passengers were a group of 41 elderly tourists anxiously looking forward to a 12-day Mediterranean cruise. Captain Victor Grubbs, the Pan Am pilot, also peered through the thick fog, as he followed the Dutch flight down the runway. At times visiblity was zero on the runway causing the Pan Am flight to taxi at barely 6 miles per hour instead of the usual 20. However, both pilots were professionals who had taken off and landed in visually impaired conditions before. Captain Van Zanten was considered KLM's top pilot and was their chief flight instructor, with 13,000 hours of flight experience under his belt.

When KLM 4805 reached the end of the runway it performed a difficult 180 degree turn and waited for the tower's permission to take off. Pan Am 1736 was to have turned off the runway onto a side taxiway, allow the Dutch flight to take off, and then continue down the runway for its own departure. The tower was waiting for Captain Grubbs's communication that they were cleared of the runway.

However, Captain Van Zanten did something that no one expected and, to this day, no one can fully explain. He began his takeoff without permission from the tower. It must have been impossible for the Dutch pilot to see through the fog before him as he rolled down the runway at close to 180 miles per hour. It wasn't until the last second that he would have seen his error. There, directly in his path, was Pan Am 1736 desperately trying to maneuver out of the path of the oncoming jet. KLM 4805 tried to pull up, but there was simply not enough time. It struck the Pan Am jumbo jet, shearing off its familiar bubble top and then slammed back into the ground and exploded into a ball of flame. In just a few seconds it was all over. All 234 passengers and the 14 crew members on the KLM plane were killed. 326 of the 378 passengers and 9 of the 16 crew members aboard Pan Am 1736 were killed. The total of 583 deaths is the highest to this day for any type of aviation disaster.

It is because of tragedies like this that aviation has very strict guidelines and rules concerning activities in and around airports. The cardinal rule is that you depend on instructions from the control tower before landing and taking off. This especially holds when the pilot is visually impaired by fog. The control tower has a perspective that the pilot just doesn't have — they can see the whole picture and can keep all the different complexities of a working airport working smoothly, reducing the chances for disastrous accidents like that at Tenerife on March 27, 1977.

Today we are living at a time when a moral fog has descended over our culture. Only a few decades ago, moral issues were considered fairly clear. Yes, there were some ambiguities here and there, but for the most part people believed they knew who they were and what their moral obligations were. Today it seems as if every old moral principle is open to question. Is it always wrong to lie or cheat? Should one abstain from sexual activities until marriage? Is homosexuality an acceptable alternative lifestyle? "Well," we are told, "it depends on the situation, or the circumstances, or the person themselves. After all, we can't be judgmental. We need to be tolerant of the beliefs and practices of others."

No area has been left untouched by the moral fog. One area where its presence has been very influential is in the practice of medicine. So many changes have occurred in medical practice in the last half of the 20th century that a whole new field has developed to act as a kind of "control tower" helping to provide guidance concerning moral issues in medicine and the life sciences: bioethics.[1]

No area has been left untouched by the moral fog.

The purpose of this book is to offer a Christian introduction to issues in bioethics. This means it is unapologetically written from a Christian perspective. The Christian perspective itself encompasses a wide range of beliefs and practices and not all Christians are going to agree on the positions this book will offer on these issues. Broadly, by the Christian perspective I mean the following: The triune God is the creator and cessionaire of the universe. Humans are created in the image of God and as such are rational beings, which makes them "morally conditioned."[2] However, this image is diminished by sin, and therefore humans are separated from fully experiencing God's love and justice. Jesus Christ is the incarnation of the second person of the trinity, fully God and fully human, who lived on earth and taught how we are to relate to God and our fellow humans. His crucifixion, death and resurrection were for the expiation of the sins of humankind and through him eternal life is offered to all who believe in him. The Scriptures are the inspired revelation of God and are authoritative concerning matters of faith and practice. The church is the institution commissioned by Jesus to spread the gospel throughout the world by being the living revelation of the love of God in an effort to call all persons to a loving relationship with God. It is this call to fellowship and union with God and Christlikeness that is the heart and soul of Christian ethics and is that which separates it from a purely secular ethic. This is the perspective from which this book plans on evaluating issues in bioethics.

What Is Causing the Moral Fog?

Let's begin by asking, "Why is modern medicine in a moral fog?" Several factors can be noted that together have put much of medical practice in a moral quagmire.

1. *The New Epidemiology*: For virtually the entire course of human history up until the middle 1800s, human beings died mainly of infectious and parasitic diseases often exacerbated by famine or epidemics. Maternal and infant mortality was high and the life expectancy was under 50. During the Civil War more soldiers died of infectious diseases and unsanitary conditions than of battle wounds. As a result specifically of that war, beginning in the mid-1800s new developments emerged in public sanitation, immunization and antiseptic techniques in childbirth and surgery. By the 1920s, with new and improved medical and surgical techniques most people began to live longer and die later in life. With the development of penicillin in the 1940s during World War II entire diseases that had long plagued mankind were all but completely eradicated. In the end, rather than infectious diseases, most people are now dying of long, drawn-out degenerative diseases: cancer, heart disease, stroke, etc. The age and pattern of the way in which we die has changed drastically in the past 100 years.

2. *The New Technology*: Along with being able to live longer, in just the past 35 years new technology has been developed to sustain life far beyond what formerly could have been; renal dialysis, transplants, pacemakers, artificial hearts, xenografting, respiratory and pulmonary support, and genetic engineering, just to name a few examples, have all contributed to increasing the lifestyle and lifespan of many persons who just a few years ago had no hope of a long life. We can even work within the environment of the womb itself to increase the chances of a struggling unborn child to survive. However, all of this technology has also contributed to drawing out the dying process itself. We can keep the lungs breathing and the heart beating for almost an indefinite period of time to the point where the very definition of death has come into question. Such treatment is not cheap. Today it is estimated that

the largest percentage of the average person's lifetime medical costs will be spent on their last week of life.

3. *The New Emphasis on Patient Autonomy and Rights*: There has been a significant shift in medical decision making in the past 40 years. Before 1970 a paternalistic and authoritarian attitude was generally adopted by most health care workers toward patients. Codes of Ethics developed before 1970 tended to emphasize the duties of health care workers rather than the rights and respect for the needs of patients. It wasn't that patient needs and desires were ignored, it was just that the doctor "knew best." His authority, as well as that of the medical community as a whole, was generally not questioned. He knew what you needed and your input would simply be "getting in the way" of his doing his job.

> *Medicine was not spared the 1960s emphasis on individual rights.*

However, In the 1960s there was a revolution concerning individual **rights**. This began in the African-American civil rights movement of the early '60s, but soon broadened to include such areas as women's rights, student rights, gay rights and others. Almost all ethical and legal issues are now being formed by the language of "rights." Medicine was not spared in this new emphasis on individual rights, and "patient rights" became one of the primary concerns of the medical community. The paternalistic medical model of times gone by has given way today to a model in which the patient becomes the primary authority in medical decisions. Over the past 20 years we have seen a growth in such areas as the right to die, the right to refuse treatment, a woman's right to her own body, the fetus's right to live, and many other areas. Codes of ethics emphasizing patient rights have sprung up such as the American Hospital Association's "Patients' Bill of Rights"

(1972) and the American Nursing Association's Code for Nurses (1976). When so many different parties are demanding their rights, there is bound to be ethical conflict.

4. *The Cultural Shift in Morality from Absolutism to Pluralistic Relativism:* Along with all the changes in medicine itself, there has been a dramatic shift in American culture in the last 40 years. The shift has been from an absolutist moral framework to a relativist framework. As an example, compare the 1950s to the 1990s. In the 1950s there was general agreement on a significant amount of moral areas. Certain things, such as lying, sexual promiscuity, divorce, pornography, were frowned upon and considered morally wrong. It wasn't just the actions; it was the attitude people generally had to morality itself — some things were wrong and some things were right and that's all there was to it. At least on the popular level, there was an almost universal agreement on morality.

In the 1990s things have changed. Those actions we once thought were wrong have all been questioned, and today it seems as if there isn't a moral issue that isn't open to debate. Again, it's not so much that our actions are different, but the significant difference is in the attitude that the average modern person has today toward morality — there are almost no things that are absolutely right or wrong any more. Morality is based purely upon personal preferences and has become extremely subjective.

> *The major cause for moral relativism*
> *is the advent of modern pluralism.*

The major cause of this **moral relativism** is the advent of modern pluralism. Pluralism is the recognition that there are in fact many different cultures each with their own separate ethical and social values. In and of itself, there is nothing new in the recognition that different culture groups often have different values. However, one of the tenets of modern pluralism is that our ideas about morality are completely dependent on the culture in which we have been raised. This is called **cultural determinism**. Modern pluralism holds that, because we are all culturally determined, no one person is in the completely objective position to judge which culture group's ethical values are the "right ones." Therefore all views must be accepted as having an equal claim to being "right."

However, it would be wrong to say that there are no absolutes in the modern pluralistic relativist framework. There is one absolute **virtue** and one absolute moral obligation. First, the absolute virtue is the virtue of tolerance. Because of pluralism, we need to develop an attitude of toleration of other views. While we may not agree with them from our perspective, we need to respect the rights of those who hold these views and adopt a position called **fallibilism**: the real possibility that our own view of morality could be wrong and other views of morality could be right. Second, the absolute obligation which flows out of the modern **pluralistic relativism** is the obligation not to harm others. This is the **minimalistic ethic** of today: "Everything is OK as long as you don't hurt others." Therefore, according to the modern view, only one moral question is ever relevant in discussions of ethical issues: Is anyone going to be harmed in this action? If no one is harmed (and intolerance is a form of harming), then the action is morally permissible. Christian ethicists Francis J. Beckwith and Greg Koukl have rightly called the 1990s a time when "our feet are planted firmly in mid-air."[3]

All of these have influenced medical practice and made ethical issues foggy. The field of bioethics emerged as a result of that fog and attempts to help provide guidance for medical practitioners and patients as they try to steer their way through it. While bioethics began primarily from a religious perspective, today it is dominated by secular ethicists and philosophers.

The Meaning and History of Bioethics

What exactly is bioethics? One way we can understand the term is to analyze its parts. *"Bio"* is a latin word which simply means "life." For example, when you study *bio*logy, you are studying about different life forms and how they operate.

The "bio" part of bioethics means that we are concerned with the "life sciences" such as medical practice, psychology, research, animal experimentation, biochemical engineering and other natural sciences as they relate to life. However, bioethics also involves a host of peripheral areas that are affected by the life sciences such as social policies like the allocation of scarce resources, or economic issues such as national health care policies.

"Ethics" deals with a host of issues involving moral decisions of right and wrong. One can define ethics as the study and analysis of the nature of morality and moral acts. Many of us immediately think of ethics as referring to some set of rules that we are supposed to obey and our condemnation of those who don't obey them. While this is certainly part of what ethics is about, there are many other issues involved in the study of ethics. In fact we can divide the study of ethics into three major branches: **Metaethics** which deals with the meaning of moral terms and moral **justification**; Ethical Systems & Theories which deals with how we derive moral theories and our moral methodology; and Applied Ethics which deals with ethics as it applies to specific disciplines such as legal ethics, business ethics, academic ethics, and bioethics.

We can define bioethics as *the analysis and study of ethical issues and problems which arise due to the interrelationship between the practice of the medical/biological sciences and the rights and values of human beings.* What do we cover in bioethics? We can reduce the study to four areas: 1) Life and Death Issues (abortion, reproductive technologies, **euthanasia, physician-assisted suicide**, etc.), 2) Clinical or Health Care Issues (informed consent, confidentiality, deception, etc.), 3) Medical Research Issues (random clinical trials, human experimentation, genetics, cloning, etc.), and 4) Social Health Care Policy (rationing health care, macroallocation and microallocation of health care, managed care, nationalized insurance programs, etc.). While this list may not be comprehensive, most issues in bioethics can be placed under one or more of these four basic areas.

While ethical controversies surrounding the practice of medicine have always existed, bioethics as a field of its own is fairly young. Not everyone is in agreement as to exactly when bioethics began. It's probably best to say that each of the four areas developed gradually over a period of several years. Medical research ethics began because of the abuses in medical experimentation in Nazi Germany before and during World War II and the subsequent Nuremburg trials in which we began to establish codes of medical ethics. Social health care issues began with the case of the first kidney dialysis machines in 1963 in Seattle, Washington, when there was more demand for the machines than they could handle and decisions had to be made concerning who would and who would not have access to them. Clinical care issues came to the forefront during the late 1960s and early 1970s as patients began to demand more control in their own health care decisions and patient rights began to become an issue. Life and death issues usually point to the Supreme Court Roe v. Wade decision in 1973 and the Karen Ann Quinlan euthanasia case in 1975 as the beginning of those types of cases.

Bioethics as a field of its own is fairly young.

Along with these foundational cases, major articles and books began to be published concerning bioethics.[4] The majority of the early writings came from the pens of Christian theologians and experts in religious ethics. Roman Catholic authors were among the first to address these issues. The Papal Encyclicals *Pacem in Terris* (1963), *Gaudium et Spes* (1965), *Humanae Vitae* (1968) and *Evangelium Vitae* (1995) establish the Catholic Church's official stance on many medical issues. Many Roman Catholic moral theologians remain among the most vocal bioethicists today such as Richard McCormick (*How Brave a New World: Dilemmas in Bioethics*, 1981), Charles Curran (*Medicine and Morals*, 1970), Germain Grisez (*Abortion: The Myths, the Realities and the Arguments*, 1970) and Edmund Pellegrino (*A Philosophical Basis of Medical*

Practice, 1981 with David Thomasma). Protestant Christian ethicists also joined in the debate, including Joseph Fletcher (*Morals and Medicine*, 1954), Paul Ramsey (*The Patient as Person*, 1970), James Gustafson (*The Contribution of Theology to Medical Ethics*, 1975) and James Childress (*Priorities in Biomedical Ethics*, 1981). Bioethics was not to remain long in the religious arena, and soon many secular authors began to write important works including Tristram Englehart (*The Foundations of Bioethics*, 1986), Robert Veatch (*A Theory of Medical Ethics*, 1981), and Daniel Callahan (*Abortion: Law, Choice and Morality*, 1970), just to name a few. One of the most influential books in the field, *Principles of Biomedical Ethics*, by Tom Beauchamp and James Childress, was published in 1977. In addition to publications, a number of bioethics organizations were being established including the Society for Health and Human Values (1968), the Hastings Center (1969), and the Kennedy Institute of Ethics (1971). By 1980 bioethics was a well-established and respected field. In 1983 the field was officially recognized when President Reagan established the President's Commission for the Study of Ethical Problems in Medicine and Biomedical and Behavioral Research. Today there are several bioethics organizations, journals, hundreds of books, and many universities offer undergraduate and graduate degrees in bioethics.

Moral Justification

To be able to discuss the issues in this book, we need to know a little about how ethics is done and how an **ethical theory** is established. The best place to start is with moral justification.

What do we mean by justification? Everybody has beliefs about things. Our beliefs range from significant life-impacting beliefs like our belief in God to small unimportant beliefs like what they will serve for lunch today in the school cafeteria. A belief is justified when one has good reasons to maintain that particular belief. For example, your belief in God might rest on reasons like his being the best explanation for the origin of the universe or because he has touched your life in some significant way. One's belief that they are serving pizza in the school cafeteria today might be based on a reason like, they always serve it on this day of the week, you saw them preparing it in the kitchen, or other people told you they were serving pizza today. All of these are reasons for beliefs and the citing of reasons are what we call the justification for one's belief.

Not all reasons are necessarily good ones. They have to be related to the belief in a special way which we call an **inference**. This means that they "lead one" to the belief that one has, or another way of putting it is that the belief "follows" from the reasons. For example, if I said that I believed they were serving pizza today because I am married and have three children, that would not be a good reason because being married and having children has nothing to do with what they are serving for lunch in the school cafeteria. A good reason has two criteria: it is true and it infers the belief. If one has good reasons for one's beliefs, then the belief is considered a justified one.

> *A moral justification is the offering of good reasons for the moral beliefs we hold.*

A moral justification is the offering of good reasons for the moral beliefs we hold. Our moral beliefs are often formulated in a moral judgment. A moral judgment is a belief we have concerning the rightness or wrongness of a particular act. The kind of ethics in which we make moral judgments is called **normative ethics**. "Stealing money from the collection plate is wrong" is an example of a moral judgment. Every moral belief is subject to the rational challenge which is simply the question, "Why do you believe that is true?" Our answer to that question will be our moral justification. So, the question, "Why is stealing money from the collection plate wrong?" might be answered by saying things like, "Because it doesn't belong to you" or "the church needs that money to meet its needs" or "that is not how Jesus would want us to live." All of these are reasons we might cite to support our judgment that stealing from the collection plate is wrong.

When we are asked to give a justification for our moral beliefs by citing the reasons we call this a moral argument. We need to be careful because "argue" can mean a couple of things. Usually when we think of an argument we mean an emotional fight between two persons that often ends up in hurt feelings. That is not what is meant here. An argument is another word for justification and is simply the citing of reasons for beliefs we regard to be true. All arguments have three parts: **premises** (the reasons), a conclusion (the belief we hold), and the relationship between the premises and conclusion (the inference). In morality we formulate moral arguments to arrive at our conclusion or belief which is formed as a moral judgment.

As we present reasons for a particular moral judgment, it is common to appeal to higher levels of justification to support our particular moral judgment. In other words, the rational challenge can be raised concerning our reason and then the reason itself needs to be justified. As we continue to justify further reasons, we tend to become more general or abstract. We can point to at least four basic levels of justification: judgments, rules, principles, and theories.[5]

Suppose you know of a situation where a teacher, Professor Keith, tells a lie to one of his students, Wayne, concerning a class assignment that Wayne needs to do in order to pass the course Professor Keith is teaching. You might formulate the following moral **judgment**: "It was wrong for Professor Keith to lie to Wayne concerning that assignment." Notice that the moral judgment is very specific about a very specific act. There is an indefinite number of possible moral situations and therefore an indefinite number of moral judgments as well. Now suppose a friend of yours asks you *why* that specific act was wrong. You would likely justify your judgment by appealing to a higher level to show why it is wrong. The next level up is generally the **rule** level. Rules are guidelines established concerning how actions are to be performed within a particular context. Different contexts have different rules. For example, in this context you might say, "It is wrong because teachers have a professional obligation to be honest with students concerning course requirements." Note how we are still fairly specific, we are speaking in terms of a specific profession and its obligations, and yet we are not as specific as on the judgment level. Instead of speaking of a specific teacher in a specific situation we are now speaking of all teachers in all situations similar to that of Professor Keith. While there may be a lengthy list of rules governing types of behaviors, there are not nearly as many rules as there are judgments. Rules can often be found in professional codes of ethics.

The difference between rules and principles might not be too clear at first glance.

However, suppose your friend continues to push the issue and now asks the rational challenge of why we have this rule in the teaching profession. The next level you might appeal to would be the **principle** level. The difference between rules and principles might not be too clear at first glance. The way I am using them here, rules are context specific, while principles are general, overriding moral guidelines that apply across a spectrum of different contexts. We can derive our rules from these overriding moral principles. While there may be debate about rules and their application, principles seem to be more generally recognized by most rational persons. For example, you might justify the rule concerning teachers' obligations to be honest with students as an application of the principle of respect for a person's **autonomy or dignity**. Respect for autonomy or dignity means recognizing that persons have the freedom to make choices concerning decisions and treating them in such a way as to allow them to freely make their choices. However, if they do not have accurate information, their ability to choose will be impeded. Therefore to lie to someone disrespects their autonomy and dignity. When we get to this level, we are speaking on much more general terms than rules, and there are really only a handful of ethical principles.

However, if challenged, what do we base our moral principles on? This takes us to the highest level in normative ethics, the ethical **theory**. An ethical theory is an entire system of ethical principles coherently related to one overriding maxim which is established external to normative ethics itself. It is usually based on a particular worldview about the nature of goodness. For example, if one believes that goodness is a particular state of affairs, like being happy, then one's ethics will be based on what makes one happy. If one believes that goodness is found in the nature of God, then his or her theory will be based on what reflects God's nature. At this level we are extremely abstract and we find very few actual ethical theories. What happens if we are challenged at this level? At this point we would need to step outside of the area of normative ethics and defend our entire worldview. Such a step is outside the scope of this book. However, as I stated earlier, this book is written from the Christian perspective or worldview. Therefore our ethical theory will be a reflection of that worldview.

How far does one realistically need to go in justifying one's moral beliefs? In general, the level in which you cease to justify is that where agreement can be found or where one feels he or she has adequately supported his or her beliefs. For example, if you and your friend agree with the accepted professional ethics of teachers, then there is no need to justify one's moral beliefs further about the wrongness of Professor Keith's actions. However, if you or your friend have further questions, you need to explore the higher levels of moral justification, including your ethical theories. It is to those theories that we now turn.

Ethical Theories

Perhaps the best way to approach our discussion of ethical theories is to analyze what is involved in any moral event. I would propose there are at least three things involved: a *person* doing an *act* that has certain desired *results*. The major ethical theories I want to examine ground themselves in one of these three aspects of a moral event. For some people, the most important aspect of a moral action is the result. What makes an act a good moral act is that it achieves a good result. This view is called *consequentialism*. For others, certain acts are simply right or wrong in and of themselves regardless of the results. For example, truthtelling is good no matter what the results are. This view, which concentrates on the rightness or wrongness of the act, is called *deontology*. Finally, there are those who say that the primary emphasis in ethics should not be on the acts or results, but on what kind of person we are. The goal is to become persons of high character or virtuous persons. If we become good persons, the actions and results will follow. This view is called *virtue ethics.* I wish to examine each of these three views in detail.[6]

For the consequentialist, the primary emphasis in determining if an act is right or wrong is the consequences or results of the action. Take lying for example. For the consequentialist, lying is usually wrong because it usually produces bad consequences, like mistrust between persons. Trust is necessary for relationships to succeed, therefore trust is good. To lie usually betrays this goodness. Therefore lying is usually wrong. However, if lying can produce a good result, then it would not be wrong. If I need to lie to save someone's life, that is a good result and lying would not be wrong in that case. Therefore lying is not always wrong, it depends on the consequences. The consequentialist might even believe that it is *usually* wrong, but not *absolutely* wrong. There are no absolute rights or wrongs for a consequentialist, at best all he can offer are general rules of thumb based on past experience with the usual results of our actions. If this sounds like "end justifies the means" thinking, that is exactly what it is. In fact, the consequentialist will tell you that the only thing that justifies the means is the end.

Consequentialism

There are two ethical theories that are consequentialistic. If you are talking about the ultimate consequences for me, that theory is called *Egoism*. If you are talking about the consequences for everybody, that theory is called *Utilitarianism.*

1. *Egoism.* Egoism itself can be broken into two types: **psychological egoism** and **ethical egoism**. Psychological egoism says that all our actions are ultimately done out of our own self-interest. It claims that we have no choice, we have to act ultimately for self. If we do a beneficial act for someone else, we are really doing it just to fulfill our own desires. They would point to such things as the good feelings we get when we do good things or the reputation we have for doing something good as the real reasons why we do good actions for others. We may think we are doing it for someone else, but we are just deceiving ourselves because we are really doing it for self. A completely **altruistic** act (one done totally for the welfare of another) is simply impossible according to this theory. An early proponent of psychological egoism was the British philosopher Thomas Hobbes (1588-1697).

> *I may do many actions that are not ultimately in my self interest.*

While psychological egoism does seem to have some truth to it and many actions we do are to fulfill our own desires, there are some serious problems with it. First, there are many actions that I may do that are not ultimately in my self interest but, because of temptation, I do them anyway. Examples are sinful acts or smoking. Second, psychological egoism doesn't seem to recognize that there may be nonintentional by-products to my actions that have nothing to do with their morality. We morally judge actions by **intentions** and motivations. For example, if you are driving in the rain and need to signal for a left turn with your hand (because your turn signal is broken), you may realize you are going to get your hand wet. However, your intention or aim is not to get your hand wet, it is to signal a turn. Getting your hand wet is an unintended by-product of your action, even though it was foreseeable. No one would say that the intended reason you stuck your hand out the window was to get it wet. In the same way, though it is true that I may get personal satisfaction out of helping others, that satisfaction can merely be a by-product of my intended action to help others. Finally, psychological egoism is not saying that I normally act out of self interest, it says it is impossible for me to act otherwise. However, no evidence is offered to support this claim. No matter how much a person claims his or her action was altruistic, the psychological egoist will merely assert that it was egoistically motivated. An assertion is not an argument. They really have no way to prove the theory at all, so it remains an unprovable assertion.

Ethical egoism differs from psychological egoism in that it claims that we *ought* to act in a manner that ultimately serves our best interest. This theory recognizes that it is possible to do an altruistic act, but in fact one never should. The use of the word "ultimate" is important here. It means that I may do actions from which others benefit, but ultimately I do it because it serves my self-interest. Those who hold this view often say that this would produce the best kind of world — if everybody looks out for themselves all will benefit. This is the basis of a capitalistic economic system. As a businessman, I am looking out for my own profits, so I will build a better mousetrap than the next guy. Someone else will come along and, looking out for his profits, will try to build a better one yet. The result is that society benefits with an excellent mousetrap because of the competitive spirit a free market economy engenders. This was the classic argument of the economist and philosopher Adam Smith (1723-1790). One of the most well-known modern proponents of ethical egoism was Ayn Rand (1905-1982).

However, ethical egoism also has some serious problems. First, it is difficult to believe that all will benefit if we are only looking out for ourselves. What happens when our interests conflict? If my ethics is based solely on looking out for myself, no moral rules exist to keep me from doing cruel or unjust actions to others, or them to me. Second, if my primary justification for ethcial egoism is that it is best for everyone, then I am not really arguing for egoism but for utilitarianism. Third, I have to hope that no one else becomes an egoist, for they might use it against me. Therefore I can never share with someone that they should become an ethical egoist, for it could be self defeating if they use it against me — I would not be doing that which was ultimately in my best interest. However, if I believe ethical egoism is the right view of accomplishing the good, but can't promote it to others, then many recognize there is a problem with it as an ethical theory. A key aspect of an ethical theory is that it promotes the good. Fourth, if ethical egoism is true, how are we to evaluate the death of Christ? We would have to say that either he did it ultimately for himself or he was morally wrong. Yet Scripture is clear many times that he "gave his life as a ransom for many" (Mark 10:45; see also John 3:16; 10:15; Eph 5:25; 2 Cor 5:19).[7] Finally, we often speak of good moral acts as praiseworthy. Yet there is something counterintuitive in praising someone for doing something that he ultimately just did for himself. Therefore, I believe both forms of egoism have enough problems that they should be abandoned as ethical theories.

How are we to evaluate the death of Christ?

2. *Utilitarianism.* Utilitarianism is the consequentialistic theory that says the morally right thing to do is that which provides the greatest happiness to the greatest number of people. This is called the utility principle. Two philosophers are primarily responsible for this theory: Jeremy Bentham (1748-1832) and John Stuart Mill (1806-1873). It is one of the most well-known ethical theories in the history of ethics and is one of the most popular today. This is especially true in modern American society where we hold that the majority rules in decision making. That is what utilitarianism says — whatever makes the majority happy is the right thing to do. Some utilitarians want to broaden "happy" to mean a number

of things: fulfilled, contented, meaningful. Utilitarianism puts together three ideas. First, one should strive to create the greatest balance of good over evil. They recognize that rarely is any single action totally good or evil, but usually a mixture. For every good thing you do, there are other good things you are not doing, and whenever a good thing is not done, we call that evil. Therefore you should choose to do those actions that have a greater balance of good over evil. This is called **proportionalism**. Second, utilitarians identify good with happiness and evil with pain. Finally, they recognize that happiness should be spread as widely and as equally as possible, again with the recognition that rarely will everyone be happy. Some utilitarians apply the utility principle to each situation independent of other situations or general guidelines. "What will produce the greatest happiness to the greatest number in this specific situation itself?" This is called **act utilitarianism**. Other utilitarians believe that general rules can be formed which usually provide the greatest happiness for the greatest number of people and that these rules can guide one in each situation he encounters. These are called **rule utilitarians**.

How do you measure happiness?

Critics of utilitarianism cite a number of problems with the view. First, how can one measure the "amount" of happiness and compare it with some other "amount" of happiness that may be so different as to make them **incommensurable**? Jeremy Bentham actually attempted to measure happiness by creating a unit of happiness which he called a "hedon" and a calculus for measuring happiness. However, such ideas are foolish. Who is happiest: a child who received the toy he really wanted for Christmas, a bride on her wedding day, or the elderly woman who just found a liver is available for her transplant? There is just no way to comparatively measure happiness. Second, should happiness be the goal of morality?

Isn't there more to life than just being happy. If I could offer you a pill which would make you happy, but would also make you severely retarded so that you could never accomplish anything in life but would be a vegetable, would you take it? Most people recognize that happiness shouldn't always be the ultimate goal of our lives. Third, under utilitarianism certain goods like persons, truthfulness, and even morality itself end up having extrinsic value and not intrinsic value. They only have value if they produce some social utility, but have no value in and of themselves. Suppose that, in order to provide the greatest happiness for the greatest number, we would have to sacrifice an innocent person. Utilitarianism would be forced in saying that such a sacrifice would be appropriate. But then what are we saying about that person? We are saying that their only value is in providing social utility. Fourth, under this view the minority always suffer for the sake of the majority. Unfortunately in our society this often ends up being the same group of people. Who is looking out for their desires? Finally, can we really know what the consequences of our actions will be? When we drop a pebble into a pond we simply do not know where the ripples will travel or what they will touch. If we cannot know what the ultimate consequences of our actions will be, how can we use consequences as our primary guide for our ethical actions?

Both types of consequential theories hold that the primary emphasis in ethics should be on achieving good results. For the egoist, good results are ultimately what is in his or her own best interest. For the utilitarian, good results are what produces the greatest happiness for the greatest number of people. We now move to a theory which says that morality has nothing to do with results at all.

Deontology   Deontology is the view that looks at our actions and declares them right or wrong in themselves. For the deontologist lying is always a wrong and no consequences, even good ones, can ever make lying good. The deontologist thinks of morality in terms of duty or obligation. I have some things I am morally obligated to do, like tell the truth, and some things I am obligated not to do, like lie. Therefore, most deontologists believe in ethical absolutes — things are absolutely right or wrong.

However, many deontologists recognize the possibility for ethical obligations to conflict. For example, it is possible that I might be faced with a moral dilemma in which I am obligated to perform two moral duties which are in conflict — if I do one I can't do the other. For example, lying to save a life. I am obligated not to lie, but I am also obligated to save life. How do I handle such a situation? Some deontologists recognize that my duties are not absolute in the extreme sense, but are *prima facie* duties. *Prima facie* means literally "at face value." *Prima facie* duties are moral obligations that hold in normal cases unless they conflict with stronger obligations, in which case they can be overridden by the stronger obligation. They are "absolute" in normal cases where there is no conflict. However, they are not absolute only in the rare case where another more fundamental duty comes into conflict. This view has also been called qualified **absolutism**.

There are three different ethical theories that are deontological in their approach to ethics. Their difference lies, for the most part, in where they obtain their duties.

Christians would point to the Bible as the authoritative basis of God's commands.

1. *Divine Command Theory.* This ethical theory proposes that our ethical duties are grounded in the commands of God. Since commands are always verbal, this means that one has to have some form of verbal divine revelation to inform one of God's commands. This revelation is the authoritative basis for all ethical duties. Christians would point to the Bible as the authoritative basis of God's commands. Examples would be the 10 Commandments as well as the commandments of Jesus and the moral instructions which are scattered throughout the

New Testament epistles. Some of these are explicit commands while others are models of how one should morally respond to a given situation. An important early proponent of this theory of ethics was William of Occam (c.1285-1389) while modern proponents have been Robert Adams and Glen C. Graber.

For many Christians this may seem like the correct ethical theory, however it has some problems. Before commenting on the problems with this view I want to make it clear that I am not denying that the Bible is the authoritative Word of God, nor am I denying that it contains authoritative moral instruction. As a Christian myself I believe firmly that Scripture is the inspired and authoritative Word of God. However, I do believe there are some problems with basing one's ethical theory solely on the commands of God. I see at least three problems with this view. First, one has to make a choice between different writings that claim to be the Word of God and yet are incompatible. Islam claims that the Koran is the Word of God. Yet the Koran and the Bible are incompatible in several areas. For example, the Bible teaches a man may marry only one woman at a time (Gen 1:27; Matt 19:4-6; 1 Tim 3:2,12) but the Koran allows for a man to have up to four wives at a time (Sur II:3). Since they are mutually incompatible, many would argue that they cannot both be the Word of God. Therefore the divine command theorist will first have to justify why his revelation is the depository of God's commands.

There are different writings that claim to be God's word, but are incompatible.

Second, what about those who do not have this divine revelation in their possession? What are they to base their ethical theory on if they do not have the commands of God? Some might point to natural revelation, but the **divine command theory** does not give you that option — commands are verbal instructions and you cannot get them by looking at nature. Can we hold those who were not given the commands responsible for keeping them if they never had them? Would it be fair if I made my students responsible for an assignment that I had never told them about?

However, the most significant problem with the divine command theory is that it reduces to **voluntarism**. Voluntarism is the view that morality is based on the will of God. In other words, what makes something good is that God simply wills it so. This is an ancient problem that even Plato addressed in his book *Euthyphro*. The problem is that if morality is just whatever God wills, then it is possible that God could have willed something evil, like child abuse, to have been good. But then that seems to make morality purely arbitrary — like God is flipping a coin to decide what is right and wrong. Also, how would a voluntarist answer the question "Is God good?" If good is "what God wills" then how do we know if God is good? The other horn of the dilemma is that if we say that God cannot will something bad to be good, then there is a standard he has to answer to outside of himself, morality. But if God has to answer to something outside of himself, how can he be the "supreme" being? Many have pointed the way out of this mess by abandoning voluntarism altogether, and opting for a view called **essentialism**. This view says that morality is not based on the *will* of God, but on the *nature* of God. Morality is derived from his very essence. This means that God is not free, but that he is limited by his nature. Scripture affirms this position when it says God cannot lie (Num 23:19; Titus 1:2; Heb 6:18). If one is abandoning volutarism, then one needs also to abandon the divine command theory as well.

2. *Natural Law Theory*. A second deontological theory is **natural law theory**. This theory has been around for many years and is traceable back to the Stoic philosophers of ancient Greece. Aspects of it can be found in Aristotle (383-321 BC), and it was given full expression in the writings of Thomas Aquinas (1225-1274).[8] Natural law holds that all men have a built-in capacity in their human nature to distinguish right and wrong. The basic idea of natural law is that

everything that exists has a **nature** and the purpose of all things are to function in accordance with that nature. This is called the **teleological view of creation**: God designed creation to function a certain way. He provided rational laws in order for creation to function appropriately. Natural objects like trees and rocks function according to physical laws and nonhuman animals according to the laws of instinct within their species. However, humans are made in the image of God and this sets them apart in two ways. First, they have the freedom to choose to follow the natural law or not. Second, the essence of their nature is their ability to reason and reflect about things. This means they have the ability to discover through reason and reflection those moral norms which will lead them to live in accordance with their nature. Natural law is not based on reason, but on our human nature. It is discoverable through reason and reflection. The moral laws discovered through natural law are universal and eternal and can be known by all through reason and reflection. They can also be used to judge individuals, societies, and human civil laws. Civil laws or individual behaviors that are not in accord with natural law are considered ethically impermissible. Finally, it is important to note that natural law does not discount the need for Scripture. Christian natural law theorists agree that natural law is not sufficient when it comes to man's relationship with God, and special divine revelation is needed for certain truths such as man's sinfulness and the need for God's grace in providing salvation. Natural law does not teach that man can earn merit before God apart from his grace. However, there is a correspondence between the moral norms of Scripture and those discoverable through natural law. Natural law never contradicts a moral norm of Scripture.

Moral laws determined by natural law are universal and eternal and are known by reason and reflection.

Natural law has its critics, and they have raised some serious problems. First, with the advent of Darwinian evolution, many seriously question the teleological view of creation proposed by natural law. If evolution is true, nothing in nature has a purpose. Everything is just chance and random selection. Therefore there are no laws guiding creation and man does not have a specific way he is supposed to function. Second, some question the idea of man having a universal and unalterable nature which he shares with all men. Some would say there are no such things as "natures" at all, only particular things with similar features. This would mean that each thing is a law unto itself; there are no universal laws. There is no set way a thing is "supposed" to function. Others believe, that while there is a human nature, it changes between cultures or individuals. Finally some argue that natural law is trying to create an *ought* from an *is*. Just because man is a certain way, doesn't imply he ought to be that way. How one answers these objections will depend on one's view of evolution and "natures." If one rejects Darwinian evolution and accepts that a divine creator designed the world so that things have "natures" and are to function according to a certain manner, then these objections seem to lose their force. Sometimes arguing an "ought" from an "is" is possible. If the definition of a watch is that it is an object that accurately tells time, then we can say that because of what it "is," it "ought" to accurately tell time. If it doesn't, then we can justifiably say that it is not functioning properly. In the same manner, if a person is designed to live according to a particular nature, and he doesn't, then he is not functioning properly. Natural law helps man to function properly.

3. *Kantian Deontology* A third type of deontology is **Kantian deontology** and it is perhaps the most well known of the deontological views. Many consider Immanuel Kant (1724-1804) as the most influential modern philosopher to have lived. This is certainly true in the area of epistemology, or philosophy of knowledge. However he was also influential in developing a deontological ethic based on pure rational

thought. Kant began by rejecting any sort of ethics based on consequences. If one depends solely on consequences, what will keep one from doing the wrong if it produces desirable consequences? He also rejected any ethics based on "natural inclinations." What Kant meant here were emotions like love, compassion, pity, patriotism, and the like. For example, some might feed the poor because they have compassion on them. However, reasoned Kant, what would motivate us to feed the poor if we didn't have such feelings? One cannot base one's ethic on emotions. Only one **motive** counts for Kant, duty. He calls this "the good will": to do right for no other reason than because it is right. That is the only motive that matters. Kant is very strict as to what counts as a moral act and what doesn't. For Kant, if you do an act out of compassion or to achieve certain consequences, you may be acting in accordance with duty, but you are not acting out of duty and therefore you are not doing a good moral act.

If everyone lied, no one would assume anyone was being honest.

According to Kant, how do we determine the right thing to do? Here he gives us one of the most famous statements in all philosophy, the **categorical imperative**. Kant formulated the categorical imperative several ways, but the one that is most well known is: "Act according to that maxim by which you can, at the same time, will that it should be a universal law." In other words, if you want to know if an action is right or wrong, universalize it so that everybody can do it. What would happen? Take lying: what if everybody lied? "Well," we might say, "that would produce disastrous consequences." Is that what Kant means? No, because that would just make him a consequentialist and, as we saw, he rejects consequentialism. What Kant means is that it would be irrational because in universalizing lying, you defeat the very reason why lying works. The only reason lying works is because people assume you are being honest. But if everyone lied, no one would assume anyone was being honest. The very act of universalizing the lying, defeats lying. So the act of lying becomes self defeating when we universalize it and that is irrational. Kant thought this method of universalizing can help anyone determine if any act is right or wrong. In that sense he believed he had a truly rational ethic.

Kant has not been without his critics. First, many have been critical of Kant because he does not seem to allow for exceptions to our moral duties. He is an unbending absolutist in his view of morality. However, what happens if moral duties conflict? Kant does not seem to recognize this possibility and provides no way out of true moral dilemmas. It took another deontologist, W.D. Ross, to come up with the concept of *prima facie* duties we mentioned above. Second, there are some who have pointed out problems with Kant's method of universalization. Suppose we act according to the maxim, "Telemarketers should be exterminated." It doesn't seem to be self-defeating to universalize this maxim. In fact if one really hates telemarketers, there doesn't seem to be anything wrong with this maxim. There is no irrational contradiction here as Kant supposes there would be. We can also do the opposite, universalize nonmoral maxims like, "whenever one is in the shower, one sings" without contradiction. However, this does not make this morally obligatory just because it is universalizable. Finally, Kant is criticized because of his strong insistence that the only acceptable motive for an act to be considered is duty and his absolute rejection of consequences and emotions. Can one simply ignore consequences the way Kant suggests? If my moral duty results in hundreds dying, should I simply ignore that? While consequences may not be an adequate basis for one's moral theory, one does not have to ignore them altogether. The same can be said for emotions. Most ethicists agree that there is something wrong with a person who does not feel compassion at the suffering of another human being and then act to relieve that suffering out of compassion. Yet for Kant such emotions have no moral value at all. The problem with "duty" is that it simply fails to inspire and motivate most persons to moral action.

We have looked at three deontological theories. While they are different in some respects, they all have at least one thing in common: they believe moral acts are intrinsically good. This intrinsic goodness may derive from different grounds. For the Divine Command Deontologist the intrinsic goodness of acts is grounded in the will of God. For the Natural Law Deontologist the intrinsic goodness of acts is grounded in the nature of God of which our nature is a reflection. For the Kantian Deontologist the intrinsic goodness of acts is grounded in the reason of man. We now move to a theory that says the consequentialist and deontologist have totally misplaced the debate by emphasizing what we do, instead of who we are.

Virtue Ethics

The theories we have concentrated on thus far have one thing in common: they have concentrated on the right thing to do in a given moral situation. We now turn to a system that believes it lifts ethics to a higher plain. Virtue ethics is not concerned so much with what we do, but the kind of person we should be. It is the view that morality should be conceived as primarily concerned, not with acts or consequences, but with the cultivation of moral virtues or traits of character. The emphasis is placed on the character of the person as primary in evaluating and performing moral actions. A true moral act has its basis in a virtuous characteristic. The primary purpose of ethics is to develop virtuous persons. This view is among the oldest in the history of ethics, going all the way back to Plato (427-347 BC) and Aristotle (383-321 BC) as well as being adopted by many of the early church fathers, including Augustine (AD 354-430) and by Thomas Aquinas in the medieval period. It fell out of favor during the enlightenment, but has recently seen a tremendous resurgence.

What is a virtue? The word "virtue" is equivalent to the Greek word *arete* meaning "excellence." Excellence always implied the idea of functioning well and appropriately on a regular basis: a knife's virtue was that it was sharp, a horse's virtue was its speed. In the moral sense, a virtue is a trained behavioral disposition to continually live in a good and righteous manner, a manner of moral excellence. By a "trained behavioral disposition" we mean something like a habit. A habit is something we learn through practice and repetition. We get so accustomed to it that it is like second nature to us — we don't really have to think about it much to do it. Take driving a car: When you first learn to drive you carefully pay attention to every detail of what you are doing. However, after years of driving, we often don't even think about what we are doing; we drive by habit. It becomes a part of us. Virtues are like that. We practice living a certain way until it becomes a part of our character. Virtuous persons are often described as men or women of integrity, courage, fairness, humility, diligence, and a host of other virtuous characteristics. It is more than just doing good acts, these morally admirable traits have become a part of the person we are. This doesn't make us perfect, but it makes us consistent. If you knew a man of integrity, and heard from someone that he wasn't honest in a particular situation, your first thought might be, "That doesn't sound like him. It is out of character for him to act that way." That is how virtues are supposed to work.

> *Virtue ethics is concerned with the kind of person we should be.*

Virtue ethics holds that we are supposed to be developing continually into virtuous persons, aspiring every day to be better. We are not supposed to be struggling all our lives with the same vices or sins. We should overcome them and move on to other mountains to scale. Nobody is born virtuous, all need to acquire the virtues through training and practice. For example, suppose there are two students who both have an opportunity to cheat on an exam. Albert struggles with the temptation quite a while, and almost gives in to it, but finally decides not to cheat. Meanwhile, Lori doesn't even consider the option. She is aware of the opportunity, but never gives it a serious thought. While virtue ethicists admire Albert for not giving in, they would say that our goal is to become like Lori. We should become people to whom vices are not a temptation. They also recognize that this is an ethic of aspiration, and therefore is more often the goal than the realization.

Another important characteristic of virtue ethics is how we learn the virtues. Rather then appealing to lists of rules, the virtues are learned by modeling virtuous persons. These can be important people of the past and present, such as Jesus, Socrates, Gandhi, or Mother Theresa, or it could be someone intimately related to one such as a parent, relative, teacher, or a friend. Usually the virtuist will study the life of the person and get to know them as well as possible. They will approach moral situations by asking "What would he or she do in this situation?" and attempt to emulate the person.

There is no one set list of all the virtues and many people have listed many attributes as virtues. Historically, handed down from the ancients, were the seven cardinal virtues. This included the four moral virtues: prudence (practical wisdom in living life), temperance (appropriateness in the use of the passions), fortitude (the courage needed to overcome obstacles as one grows), and **justice** (fairness and equity in dealings with others). To these were added the theological virtues that applied to one's relationship with God: faith, hope and love. They believed that all other virtues flowed out from these seven.

Virtue ethics has much to commend it. It provides the motivational component missing in the "duty" based ethics of Kant and other deontologists. It recognizes that there is more to ethics than consequences because we all admire those who, like Mother Theresa, continually live in a virtuous manner, even though they do not often see good results of their work. Also, unlike Kant, virtue ethics recognizes this importance of emotions in ethical reasoning and encourages compassion and love as motivations for moral actions. Virtue ethics also provides a foundation, a developed moral character, to support us when we encounter difficult moral decisions or dilemmas.

Some sort of rule theory is needed to supplement virtue theory.

However, virtue ethics also has some problems. As nice as the virtues are, many have pointed out that they do not give us enough guidance in making decisions in specific ethical situations. It simply remains too abstract and is not practical enough. When I encounter a tough decision, it is often not enough to tell me to be a person of integrity. A second and related problem has to do with judging a person's actions as right and wrong. What if in performing an evil action a person displays one or more moral virtues? Suppose a person breaks into your house at night and sneaks right up to your nightstand while you are sleeping and takes your valuables. He is obviously exhibiting great courage. Suppose he is robbing you to feed his starving family, then he is also exhibiting great loyalty. These are good virtues, so do they now make stealing virtuous? If not, then how do we judge the action as morally wrong if all we have are virtues? It seems some sort of rule theory is needed to supplement virtue theory in order for it to work.

How should we, as Christians, appraise these theories? We have seen that they all have problems. That is usually the case in most areas of philosophy. What we often have to opt for is the theory that has the best explanatory value. In other words, it explains things best with the least amount of problems. Which theory does that from the Christian perspective? It would have to be a theory that honors God and is reflective of his nature, plan, and desires.

A Christian Appraisal of the Ethical Theories

I would like to suggest that rather than any one theory, a pluralism of theories best accomplishes that goal. We stated above that there are at least three things involved in a moral event: a *person* doing an *act* that has certain desired *results*. All three of these aspects are important, but not in the same way or at the same level. Therefore though our ethical theory is pluralistic, it needs to be properly prioritized. It seems to me that the most important aspect is the person himself or herself, and therefore I believe virtue ethics should receive first priority in a Christian ethical theory. God is much more concerned with us than he is with our actions or our accomplishments. He did not create us just to do good works or accomplish good results. Nor did he send his Son to die on the cross for our works or accomplishments. He loves us, created us in his image and wants us to fellowship with him. Therefore, it seems to me that God is primarily concerned with the kind of person we are, and that is what virtue ethics emphasizes.

The New Testament emphasis is on who you are.

This is what one observes in the New Testament. The emphasis is on who you are rather than your acts and accomplishments. Romans 12:2 says we are not to be conformed to this world, but we are to be transformed into a different kind of person. Paul picks up this theme again in Ephesians 4:24 when he admonishes us to "put on the new self, created to be like God in true righteousness and holiness" (NIV), a theme he repeats in Colossians 3. Also, we find in the New Testament an emphasis on modeling oneself after Jesus or Paul. Paul writes in 1 Corinthians 11:1, "Follow my example, as I follow the example of Christ" (NIV). Other passages emphasize the idea of modeling Christ (2 Thess 3:7-9; 1 Pet 2:21; Phil 2:5).

However, none of this discounts the need for action-guiding rules. As we saw in our discussion above, virtue ethics is inadequate by itself. We often need specific guidlines, and so action-guiding rules are necessary as well as the virtues. It would seem the primary ethic is a virtue ethic, but second in priority would be a deontological ethic. Of the three we examined, the natural law ethic appears to have the best explanatory power. First, it grounds our moral norms in the nature of God while recognizing that Scripture both confirms and supplements the norms that are discoverable by reason. Second, in affirming a natural law ethic, we also acknowledge the universality of moral norms. We can apply our moral norms to all persons in relevant similar situations, for we all have the same basic human nature. Third, natural law is taught in Scripture. We are told that God has not left himself without a witness to unbelievers (Acts 14:17), that God's power and nature have been clearly seen and understood through what has been seen so that those who practice godlessness are without excuse (Rom 1:20), and that those who do not have the divine commands do by nature the things of the law because God has written the law on the hearts of all and their conscience bears witness to it (Rom 2:14-15). So there is a place for a deontological natural law ethic in supporting the virtue ethic.

There are times when we need to consider the consequences in living out our virtues.

What about consequentialism? While this is probably the weakest of all views, one should not rule out the place of consequences in our moral reasoning. They do have a consideration, though they should be given the lowest priority. There are times when we need to consider the consequences of our actions in living out our virtues. However, we need to exercise caution due to the uncertainty of the ultimate consequences of any action. I may be thinking that I am doing an act of kindness that results in an immediate good, but may not be aware of the long range consequences that may not be good.

In putting this all together, let us borrow a term from the philosopher John Rawls, "reflective equilibrium."[9] The idea of

reflective equilibrium is that as I approach a moral event, I need to continually reflect on three ideas: new information or insights the event may present, my moral judgments, and the three different aspects of my properly prioritized pluralistic ethical theory. My goal is to maintain a proper balance or state of equilibrium in my moral life: one where I am becoming more like Jesus every day. Sometimes this will mean an adjustment of my overall system to account for new information. I must be willing to reflect and change. That is what life is all about.

Methods of Bioethics   Before moving on to discussing the many issues of medical ethics discussed in this book, we need to cover one more theoretical issue. How is bioethics supposed to be done? There has been quite a bit of debate in recent years about what approach or method one should use in doing bioethics. A number of methods have been suggested, but we will again only concentrate on the three that seem to be the most influential: **Principlism, Casuistry,** and **Ethics of Care.**[10]

Principlism[11]   Principlism can best be described as a top down approach. It begins with established principles or rules and then applies them to a particular ethical situation. The principles or rules themselves are arrived through a particular ethical theory independent of any situation. Of the three methods mentioned here, principlism has been the most dominant and influential theory. It was reflected in the historical Belmont Report (1978) and has been developed and most closely aligned with Tom Beauchamp and James Childress in their influential work, *Principles of Biomedical Ethics,* now in its 4th edition (1994). I will use their model as representative of this type of method.

Beauchamp and Childress use four principles as the basis for many more specific rules governing bioethics. The *principle of **respect for autonomy*** is first, to recognize a person's capacities, including his right to hold views, to make choices, and to take actions based on personal values and beliefs. Second it involves treating persons so as to allow or to enable them to act autonomously. The principle of respect for autonomy is usually stated in a negative form called a principle of noninterference: Autonomous actions or choices are not to be subjected to controlling constraints by others.

The *principle of nonmaleficence* is the obligation to avoid harming or injuring others. This concept is one of the oldest in medical science, being found in the **Hippocratic oath**: "I will never use treatment to injure or wrong the sick." The *principle of beneficence* is the moral obligation to act for the benefit of others. More specifically, it is to act in a manner to further the legitimate interests of others. Since it is in our interest to have good health, beneficence is obligatory for those in the medical field. It involves two aspects: providing positive benefits and balancing benefits with **harm** or risk of harm.

The *principle of justice* is the maintenance of what is just by the impartial judgment of conflicting claims and the assignment of merited rewards or punishments. Justice involves fairness, just deserts, and entitlements. It assures fair, equitable and appropriate treatment in regard to what is due or owed to persons.

Beauchamp and Childress believe that these four principles are reflective of the roles and professional obligations of health care workers and that the majority of rules regarding health care can be derived from one or more of these principles. This is not done deductively, but through a process of specification of the principles to different moral situations and conflicts and by balancing the principles and rules with one another. Specification and balancing are not only useful in applying the principles, but also help when they come into conflict. For example, suppose a physician discovers that his patient has cancer and does not have long to live. The patient is about to go on a three-month cruise vacation with his family that he has been planning on for years. Should he inform the patient? Here we have a specification of two principles: the principle of respect for autonomy and the principle of nonmaleficence. Balancing occurs as the physician considers all the factors involved in deciding which principle should take priority in this case. This is how the method of principlism works.

Casuistry   In recent years principlism, which dominated the bioethics field for over a decade, has come under sharp criticism. Some of this criticism has come from within the principlist (as broadly defined) camp itself and some has come from alternative approaches. Casuistry is an alternative method to principlism that has recently undergone a revival. For many years this method of ethical reasoning had fallen into disrepute due to its propensity for petty quibbling on minute details that made little difference to anyone. However, Albert Jonsen and Stephen Toulmin, whose book *The Abuse of Casuistry* can be credited with much of the revival of this method, claim that the poor reputation casuistry has is due to abuses of it, and not to how it is supposed to function.

Casuistry can be described as a bottom-up approach.

Casuistry rejects any sort of principlistic or rule-centered approach as being alienated from actual experience, precedent, or circumstances. Instead casuists argue our moral reasoning must begin from particular concrete situations. Casuistry can be described as a bottom-up approach. It begins with the case and, rather than appealing to moral rules or principles, identifies relevant salient features in that case that are analogous to other cases. Often there are certain paradigm or landmark cases that establish the standard by which all relevant cases are measured. For example, the Tarasoff case is a landmark case dealing with justifiable infringement of a patient's confidentiality. If a casuist is dealing with a case in which infringement of confidentiality is possibly justified, he might use the Tarasoff case as a basis for his justification, rather than appealing to rules or principles. The goal is to find a consensus among all relevant cases as to the correct moral action. Eventually, if there is a wide enough consensus of similar cases, casuists will formulate rules of the proper moral action in cases like these. The big difference is that the rules do not come from a moral theory, but from cases themselves, hence the bottom-up approach.

Casuistry can be compared to case law in which the doctrine of precedent is the main methodology. As judges make rulings on issues those rulings establish precedents for further court cases and may be appealed to as authoritative on a particular point of law. This is where a casuist's use of cases differs from a principlist's use of cases. Principlists also appeal to cases, but they usually appeal to them as illustrations of a particular principle or as how to resolve conflicts between competing principles. For the casuist, the cases are sources of authority for judgments in moral reasoning. Where the major method for principlism was specification and balancing, for the casuist it is analogy: grouping cases with relevantly similar features together and arriving at a consensus. This is how casuistry works.

Ethics of Care joins casuistry in rejecting the appeal to theoretical principles and rules in resolving moral issues in bioethics. However, rather than appeal to other cases, they emphasize responsibilities within relationships as the primary methodology in discovering what our moral actions should be. Care ethics is relationship-based as opposed to principle-based or case-based. This methodology began primarily in feminist writings and the major writers have been Carol Gilligan (*A Different Voice*, 1982), Annette Baier ("What Do Women Want in a Moral Theory," 1985) and Nel Noddings (*Caring: A Feminine Approach to Ethics and Moral Education*, 1984).[12] Gilligan discovered through studies that men tended to frame ethics in terms of rights and principles of justice while women tended to frame ethics in terms of intimacy and responsibility in relationships. However, care ethicists are quick to point out that an ethic of care is not restricted to gender and can be a methodology used by either men or women.

Care ethicists challenge two major assumptions to bioethics as it has been historically conceived: the concept of impartiality and the concept of universal principles. Rather than approaching an ethical situation as an impartial observer,

Ethics of Care

attempting to remain objective, care ethicists maintain that one should become immersed in the life of the person involved, forming intimate relationships which involve trust, love, friendship and human bonding. The care ethicist believes that this allows a strong role for the emotions in ethical reasoning that theoretical principle or rule-based approaches sorely neglect. As a result of the relationship that forms, a sense of responsibility develops and this responsibility should guide one in moral decision-making apart from impartial principles or rules. We make our decisions out of responsible faithfulness to the relationship we have developed. Sometimes conflicts will develop. Just as principlists often face conflicts between principles, ethics of care must often deal with conflicting responsibilities. However, for the care ethicist, the primary issue in such conflicts is not what the health care worker does, but how his actions are performed and what relationships are promoted. This is how an ethic of care works.

Evaluation of Methods

The methodology we will adopt in this book will be basically a principlistic approach. This approach is used for two main reasons. First, it fits best with the ethical theory we have adopted above — the pluralist approach properly prioritized. In that theory we recognized the existence of certain *prima facie* universal norms and principles which we can attribute to natural law. The principles and rules often appealed to in a principlistic methodology are in many ways identical to the same universal norms. We also recognize the importance of virtues, emotions and persons as primary in ethical reflection. This meets some of the concerns of the ethic of care. Finally, the reflective equilibrium model I suggested fits right in with the specification and balancing aspect of principlism. It also allows for the influence of cases in our moral reasoning. Reflecting on new moral situations and cases we encounter and giving them a part in our moral reasoning process answers some of the concerns of the casuists.

The second reason I am adopting the principlist approach is that, while it has its share of problems, it seems to work better than the other approaches. The main problem with casuistry is that of establishing the paradigm cases. One cannot approach a case without having some value already in mind by which we then judge the facts of the case. The paradigm case does not come to us with the values already built in — they must be supplied from somewhere else. The casuist must have assumed values already in place which he brings into bearing on the case. There is nothing about the facts of infringing confidentiality itself that tell me it is wrong — I need something like a principle to inform me of its moral value.[13] As I stated above, the principlist method allows for the influence of cases in one's moral reasoning.

> *One cannot approach a case without having some value already in mind.*

The main problem with ethic of care is simply its inadequacy as a methodology. While it rightly points out the need for emotions and loyalty in moral reflection, it does not provide a real method for making moral decisions. I also believe there is a real problem with a rejection of impartiality in that it can lead to unjust situations. The fact that one person may receive care simply because they have an established relationship that another does not have smacks of bias and discrimination. While noting the need for care to play a larger part in a full moral system, one should not quickly reject the part impartial principles play. Indeed some care ethicists have come to see that a total principleless ethic is indefensible.[14]

Having now examined and established our ethical theory and our bioethical methodology, we are ready to examine some of the main issues in medical ethics from a Christian perspective and help provide a guide for modern medicine to steer through the moral fog.

Endnotes

[1]There are several terms used for the study we are about to pursue: Bioethics, Biomedical Ethics and Medical Ethics. While there are some distinctions between the meanings of these terms, for our purposes I will use them interchangeably.

[2]By "morally conditioned" I mean that humans are moral creatures able to understand and respond to the moral concepts of right and wrong. I am borrowing this term from Stanley J. Grenz, *The Moral Quest: Foundations of Christian Ethics* (Downers Grove, IL: InterVarsity, 1997), p. 212.

[3]Francis J. Beckwith and Greg Koukl, *Relativism: Feet Firmly Planted in Mid-Air* (Grand Rapids: Baker, 1998). It is not within the scope of this book to discuss problems with modern pluralistic relativism, which I believe are many. I refer the reader to Beckwith and Koukl's excellent work.

[4]It should be noted that in the list of authors that follows only their first or most important works are cited. This list is not intended to be comprehensive, but only to name a sampling of those who were among the most influential in the early days of the bioethics movement. Several more important individuals could have been listed but space only allows a select few.

[5]I am thankful to Beauchamp & Childress for their outline of this basic structure. See Tom L. Beauchamp and James F. Childress, *Principles of Biomedical Ethics*, 4th ed. (New York: Oxford University Press, 1994), p. 15.

[6]This list is not meant to be comprehensive and many theories are not being mentioned here such as feminist ethics, communitarian ethics, an ethic of rights, an ethic of care, social contract theory, existentialistic ethics and postmodern ethical theories. Some of these will be covered in other sections of this book. I believe these three views form the main views one finds today.

[7]It is true that one passage says that Christ endured the cross "for the joy set before him" (Heb 12:2). However, this may just be a statement of a by-product of his sacrificial act. It is difficult to think that Christ's intention in dying on the cross was to experience joy himself when so many passages point to his entire mission as one of saving mankind from their sins.

[8]It is important to note that neither Aristotle nor Aquinas should be considered as primarily Natural Law theorists. While their ethical system employs the natural law, they would base their theory more on the development of virtues and therefore are better characterized as virtue ethicists.

[9]John Rawls, *A Theory of Justice* (Cambridge, MA: Harvard University Press, 1971), pp. 20-21.

[10]For an excellent discussion of the main methods of bioethics I strongly urge the special issue of the *Kennedy Institute of Ethics Journal*, Vol 5, No. 3, September 1995. Unfortunately, ethics of care was not represented in that volume.

[11]The term "principlism" has a narrow usage in that it was coined by Gert and Clouser ("A Critique of Principlism," *Journal of Medicine and Philosophy* [1990]: 15:219-236) to describe the method of ethics employed originally in the Belmont Report (1978) and developed by Beauchamp and Childress.

I am using it in a broader sense of any method that operates from a top down perspective as I describe in what follows. This would include other methods besides those of Beauchamp and Childress, including Gert and Clouser's own rule-based approach.

[12]While the view was originally touted by many as being *the* "feminist ethic" recent writings have revealed that not all feminists would agree with that evaluation and some vehemently oppose it.

[13]Recently even Albert Jonsen recognized this need. See "Casuistry: An Alternative or Complement to Principles," *Kennedy Institute of Ethics Journal*, Vol 5, No. 3 (September 1995): 237-251.

[14]See Alissa Carse, "The 'Voice of Care': Implications for Bioethical Education," *The Journal of Medicine and Philosophy* (1991): 16:5-28.

References

Ethical Theories and General Ethics Sources

Beauchamp, Tom L. *Philosophical Ethics: An Introduction to Moral Philosophy*. New York: McGraw Hill, 1982.

Denise, Theodore C., Sheldon P. Peterfreund, and Nicholas P. White. *Great Traditions in Ethics*. 9th ed. Belmont, CA: Wadsworth, 1999.

Geisler, Norman L. *Christian Ethics: Options and Issues*. Grand Rapids: Baker, 1989.

Hinman, Lawrence M. *Ethics: A Pluralistic Approach to Moral Theory*. 2nd ed. Fort Worth, TX: Harcourt Brace College Publishers, 1998.

Messerly, John G. *An Introduction to Ethical Theories*. Lanham, MD: University Press of America, 1995.

Pojman, Louis P. *Ethics: Discovering Right and Wrong*. 3rd ed. Belmont, CA: Wadsworth, 1999.

Rachels, James. *The Elements of Moral Philosophy*. 2nd ed. Belmont, CA: Wadsworth, 1993.

Rae, Scott B. *Moral Choices: An Introduction to Ethics*. Grand Rapids: Zondervan, 1995.

General Bioethics Sources

Beauchamp, Tom L. and James F. Childress. *Principles of Biomedical Ethics*. 4th ed. New York: Oxford University Press, 1994.

Beauchamp, Tom L. and Leroy Walters. *Contemporary Issues in Biomedical Ethics*. 5th ed. Belmont, CA: Wadsworth, 1999.

Childress, James F. *Practical Reasoning in Bioethics*. Indianapolis: Indiana University Press, 1997.

Edwards, Rem B. and Glenn C. Graber. *Bioethics*. Orlando, FL: Harcourt, Brace and Jovanovich, 1988.

Engelhardt Jr., H. Tristram. *The Foundations of Bioethics*. New York: Oxford University Press, 1986.

Gert, Bernard, Charles M. Culver, and Danner K. Clouser. *Bioethics: A Return to Fundamentals*. Oxford University Press, 1997.

Hauerwas, Stanley. *Suffering Presence: Theological Reflections on Medicine, the Mentally Handicapped, and the Church*. Notre Dame, IN: University of Notre Dame Press, 1986.

Kilner, John F., Nigel M. de S. Cameron, and David L. Scheidermayer, eds. *Bioethics and the Future of Medicine: A Christian Appraisal*. Grand Rapids: Eerdmans, 1995.

Lammers, Stephen E. and Allen Verhey, eds. *On Moral Medicine: Theological Perspectives in Medical Ethics*. 2nd ed. Grand Rapids: Eerdmans, 1998.

Meilaender, Gilbert. *Bioethics: A Primer for Christians*. Grand Rapids: Eerdmans, 1996.

_____, *Body, Soul and Bioethics*. Notre Dame, IN: Notre Dame University Press, 1995.

Munson, Ronald. *Intervention and Reflection: Basic Issues in Medical Ethics*. 4th ed. Belmont, CA: Wadsworth, 1992.

Pence, Gregory E. *Classic Cases in Medical Ethics*. 2nd. ed. New York: McGraw Hill, 1995.

Ramsey, Paul. *The Patient as Person*. New Haven, CT: Yale University Press, 1970.

Shannon, Thomas A. *An Introduction to Bioethics*. 3rd ed. Mahwah, NJ: Paulist Press, 1997.

Special Issue: "Theories and Methods in Bioethics: Principlism and Its Critics." *Kennedy Institute of Ethics Journal*. Johns Hopkins University Press. 5:3 (September 1995).

Veatch, Robert. ed. *Medical Ethics*. 2nd ed. Sudbury, MA: Jones and Bartlett, 1997.

Websites on Ethics and Bioethics (Please note that all websites were current as of this writing. However websites are notorious for changing. There is no guarantee that all of these sites will be running when you try them.)

I. General Ethics Sites

Ethics Updates (http://ethics.acusd.edu/index.html): Best on the Web for ethical theories and issues, many lists of sources and links to other sites.

II. General Bioethics Sites

Bioethics Links (http://ccme-mac4.bsd.uchicago.edu/CCMEDocs/EthLinks) — Sponsored by the University of Chicago, a good site with several other links, lists of journals, some full text online articles and discussion topics.

Bioethics Network of Ohio (http://www.concentric.net/~edinger/BENO/BENO.HTML) — Links to several other sites, several bibliographies and databases.

Galaxy Bioethics Links (http://galaxy.tradewave.com/galaxy/Medicine/ Philosophy/Ethics.html) — A good website sponsored by Galaxy, Inc. Especially designed for professional research in many areas. Mostly a list of other sites, some value but restrictive.

Issues in Healthcare (http://www.geocities.com/HotSprings/3872/) — An excellent site with information on a host of issues: research on human subjects, euthanasia, etc. However, you have to put up with all the Geocities advertisements which pop up every time you click on a link — just close the page that has the advertisement.

MacLean Center for Clinical Medical Ethics (http://ccme-mac4.bsd. uchicago.edu/CCME.html) — sponsored by the University of Chicago — main page — lists many resources and helpful information.

Medical Ethics (http://www.mic.ki.se/Diseases/k1.316.html) — sponsored by the Koralinski Institutet in Sweden (though the information is in English). It includes a large number of links, many of which include full text online articles.

MedNet Medical Ethics Connections (http://www.sermed.com/ethics.htm) — sponsored by Service Medical MedNet Inc.; several medical resources including codes of ethics, information on advanced directives and print-able bibliographies.

MedWeb (http://www.medweb.emory.edu/medweb) — sponsored by Emory University this site contains a list of topical links in a variety of areas, some full text online articles.

National Reference Center for Bioethics Literature (http://guweb.georgetown. edu/nrcbl/) — This is the library that contains it all; it is the major source for bioethics information. Almost every journal article or book on bioethics is located here. You can get onto BIOETHICSLINE, a comprehensive database for material on bioethics here as well as many other search engines.

University of Pennsylvania Bioethics Internet Project (http://www.med. upenn.edu/~bioethic/) — Excellent site with loads of information including links to articles online. Especially good is a section called "Bioethics for Beginners."

III. Religion and Bioethics

The following sites deal with bioethics from a religious perspective. Again they will contain essays and articles on a variety of issues. While most of these are Christian sites, their inclusion here does not necessarily imply an endorsement of everything they promote or affirm.

Catholic Resources on Medical Ethics (http://cwis.usc.edu/hsc/info/newman/resources/ethics.html) — major Catholic statements on issues in bioethics sponsored by the Newman Center of the University of Southern California.

Center for Biblical Bioethics (http://www.bfl.org/CenterBB.htm) — Sponsored by Baptists for Life, this site introduces the organization and has a good article on physician-assisted suicide, but other material must be ordered from them. A good selection of material to be ordered.

The Center for Bioethics and Human Dignity (http://www. bioethix.org/) — A major evangelical organization, they have come out with many tapes, articles and books on issues in bioethics. Their site contains some information but most of it is available to members only.

Christian Medical and Dental Society Ethics Page (http://www.cmds.org/Ethics/ethics.htm) — Good page for Christian perspectives mostly on life and death issues.

Christian Medical Ethics Page (http://ccme-mac4.bsd.uchicago.edu/CCMEDocs/Christian) — Part of the University of Chicago's website, it contains a list of articles, sites and issues specifically from a Christian perspective.

US Catholic Bishops: Healthcare Guidelines (http://www.usc.edu/hsc/info/newman/resources/chc/contents.html) — Statement of National Council of Catholic Bishops on healthcare issues.

CHAPTER 2

The Second Civil War: Abortion

The Second Civil War: Abortion

Introduction
A. The Legal Situation
   1. Prior to Roe v. Wade
   2. Since Roe v. Wade
B. The Moral Arguments for and against Abortion
   1. Proabortion Arguments
      a. The Right to Privacy Argument
      b. The Quality of Life Argument
      c. The Nonperson Argument
   2. Pro-Life Arguments
      a. Introduction
      b. The Personhood Argument
         i. The Concept of Personhood
         ii. When Does Personhood Begin?
            a) The Agnostic Theory
            b) Decisive Moment Theories
               1) Conception
               2) Implantation
               3) Brain Development
               4) The Appearance of Humanness
               5) The Attainment of Sentience
               6) Quickening
               7) Viability
               8) Birth
            c) Gradualism
            d) Conclusion
C. Scripture and Abortion
D. Conclusion

2

She could not believe it. Norma McCorvey was pregnant — again. She had only been dating this guy for four months. It was not her first pregnancy. Her first daughter was born as a result of her earlier marriage. She was just 16 when she dropped out of high school and within the year was married to 24-year-old Woody McCorvey. When she told him she was pregnant, he smacked her across the room and claimed she must have been sleeping with someone else. She moved back in with her mother and worked in a bar until her daughter was born on May 25, 1965. Her mother took custody of the child and Norma moved out. Her second pregnancy was just a year later, the father was a boyfriend she only refers to as "Joe." He wanted the baby and she didn't. So when it was born, she gave it up to him for adoption, not even knowing its sex. She never saw it again. And now here it was 1969, and she was pregnant again.

However, no one wanted this baby, least of all Norma. She wanted an abortion. However, according to Texas state law at the time, abortion was only permissible to save the mother's life. Someone suggested that she tell the gynecologist that she had been raped. She tried that, but he didn't buy it. Fearful of an illegal abortion, poor, with a drug problem and alcohol addiction, Norma contacted attorney Henry McCluskey with the purpose of making adoption arrangements. However, McCluskey put her in touch with two young, ambitious lawyers: Sarah Weddington and Linda Coffee. They were looking for the perfect case to challenge the Texas law and all state laws outlawing abortions. By the time she met with them she was eight months pregnant. They told her there was nothing they could do to get this baby aborted. They asked her at that first meeting, "Would you be willing to take your case all the way to the Supreme Court?" Norma didn't know anything about law so she figured, "Yeah, let's go for it." Norma gave birth to a boy in June of 1970 and immediately gave the child up for adoption. Meanwhile Norma's lawyers, claiming that Norma had been gang raped, filed a class action suit in federal court charging that the State of Texas had infringed her civil rights, specifically her right for privacy. Arguing for the State of Texas was the Executive Assistant District Attorney, Henry Wade. To protect her privacy, Weddington and Coffee gave Norma the pseudonym Jane Roe. They won their suit against Texas. The federal court ruled that the Texas law was vague and unconstitutional. However, the State of Texas decided to appeal the federal court's ruling to the United States Supreme Court. The case was argued before the court twice, on December 13, 1971 and again on October 11, 1972. Finally on January 22, 1973, the Supreme Court rendered its verdict on the case *Roe v. Wade* and, reminiscent of the shots fired on Fort Sumter, began the second Civil War.[1]

The Legal Situation   Perhaps no other issue is as controversial or as divisive today as is the abortion issue. Just like the Civil War of the last century, it has pitted neighbor against neighbor and brother against brother. It has been the subject of editorials and sermons that rival those of the New England abolitionists and the antebellum Southern politicians. It has even been the cause of bloodshed, not just of the millions of unborn children, but of those who have performed abortions and of those who have protested their performance. Before we examine the arguments, both for and against abortion, it is important for us to understand the legal road we traveled that has brought us to where we are today.

From about the time of the Civil War through the 1960s abortion was illegal in most states save for those rare instances when the mother's life was in danger. In most states it was a misdemeanor if one had an abortion before "quickening" (when the mother first feels life) and a capital offense after quickening. The country began to take an interest in the abortion issue in 1962 with the Finkbine baby case. Shirley Finkbine was an Arizona kindergarten teacher and mother of four when she became pregnant while taking the tranquilizer thalidomide. Thalidomide was known to cause extremely deformed children if taken by pregnant women. In fact it was known as a "monster former" and was illegal in the US, but not overseas where Finkbine had gotten her prescription. Finkbine originally requested an abortion claiming it was for the "health of the mother," a fact she would later deny. Not finding a state that would grant her an abortion, she eventually traveled to Europe where she aborted an extremely deformed baby. The case received a lot of publicity and caused many to rethink their position on abortion. Soon propositions began appearing on state ballots legalizing abortions. Colorado became the first state to liberalize its abortion laws in 1967. It was soon followed by North Carolina and California where it was signed into law by then-Governor Ronald Reagan. In 1970 New York, Alaska, Hawaii, and Washington all loosened restrictions on abortion.

Meanwhile, on the other side of the country, another important case was brewing that would have tremendous ramifications on the abortion issue. In the state of Connecticut a married couple was sold contraceptives by a health clinic. However, the sale of contraceptives was against Connecticut state law. The 1879 law, which all agreed was outdated, had been challenged twice but had been dismissed due to technicalities. However, this time the law was challenged all the way to the United States Supreme Court. It was argued that the law violated a person's right to privacy. While there is no actual right to privacy in the constitution, proponents argued that the right was part of the "penumbra" of the first, ninth and fourteenth amendments. The court agreed and in 1965 ruled on *Griswold v. Connecticut* establishing that a person indeed has a constitutionally guaranteed right to privacy. With the ruling on *Griswold*, and the proabortion movements on the state level, the stage was set for *Roe v. Wade*.

In Roe v. Wade, the Supreme Court struck down all state laws outlawing abortion.

In *Roe v. Wade* (1973) the Supreme Court ruled (7-2) that the Texas law outlawing abortion was unconstitutional because it violated a woman's right to privacy as had been determined in the *Griswold* decision. In striking down the Texas law, the Supreme Court, in essence, struck down every other state law outlawing abortion. Proabortion[2] advocates are quick to point out that the court did place limits on abortion. However, as we will see, those limits can be and are often broadly interpreted. What exactly did the court say? First, states could not restrict abortion during the first two trimesters (six months) of pregnancy except for normal procedural guidelines. **Viability** was the determining factor. In 1973 viability was between 24-28 weeks and so they settled on the trimester system of dividing the pregnancy into three 3-month (13 week) periods. This meant that a woman could have an abortion for any reason during the first six months. Second, in the last trimester, the state has a right, *but no obligation*, to restrict abortions to only those cases where the mother's health is in jeopardy. In other words, states don't have to restrict any abortions. However, if states do restrict abortions, they can only restrict them for the last three months of pregnancy and even at that time, they must allow them for the sake of the mother's health. Finally, though not specifically addressed, implied in *Roe v. Wade* was that the father of the unborn and the parents of a minor have no say in this decision. The reason is that this was a privacy issue and no one can interfere with a person's constitutional right to privacy.

On the same day the *Roe* ruling was announced, the court also made public its ruling on another abortion case *Doe v. Bolton*. This has often been called *Roe's* sister case. This case concerned a Georgia couple who attempted to get an abortion but did not meet the conditions of the then-current Georgia law. The Georgia law allowed abortions only in cases where the woman's life was in danger, the pregnancy was the result of a rape, or the fetus was seriously defective. The judgment would be left to a licensed physician and needed corroboration from two other physicians. The court ruled (7-2) the Georgia law was unconstitutional because, again, it violated a woman's right to privacy. Proabortion advocates again point out that in the *Doe* case, the court recognized that a woman's right to an abortion is not absolute and that the state has an interest in protecting the health of a "potential of independent human existence."[3] However, the most important aspect of *Doe* was the broadening of the meaning of "health of the mother in jeopardy" (the restriction placed on abortions in the last trimester as per *Roe v. Wade*) to include "all factors — physical, emotional, psychological, familial, and the woman's age — relevant to the well-being of the patient. All these factors relate to health."[4] This made abortion on demand legal for the entire nine months of pregnancy, a point made by the U.S. Senate Judiciary Committee: "Since there is nothing to stop an abortionist from certifying that a third-semester abortion is beneficial to the health of the mother — in this broad sense — the Supreme Court's decision has in fact made abortion on demand throughout the prenatal life of the child from conception to birth."[5] The impact of *Roe* and *Doe* together made null and void every state's restriction of abortion and allowed abortion on demand for the entire nine months to any woman who requested it. It was not a moderate adjustment, as many pro-abortionists would claim. It was a complete upheaval of the then current legal thinking on abortion.

Doe v. Bolton broadened the meaning of jeopardy to the mother's health.

The next major Supreme Court decision concerning abortion was *Danforth v. Planned Parenthood of Missouri* (1976). In this decision the court ruled that sections of a Missouri law were unconstitutional in requiring, among other things, spousal consent for a woman getting an abortion, and a "blanket parental consent" for a minor to get an abortion. *Danforth* made explicit what was implied in *Roe*. Next, in 1977, the Supreme Court reversed a lower district court ruling in Pennsylvania in the case of *Beal v. Doe* concerning Medicare payments for **nontherapeutic abortions**. **Therapeutic abortions** are those that are necessary for the health of the mother while nontherapeutic abortions are those which are for convenience's sake, by far the most common reason for abortions in this country. The lower court ruled that nontherapeutic abortions should be paid for by the government-funded Medicaid program. The Supreme Court stated that such payments were not required, reasoning that a negative right of noninterference in a woman's private decision did not necessarily lead to a positive right of providing benefits to her.[6]

In 1983, the Court ruled on *City of Akron v. Akron Reproductive Health, Inc.* It would be the last of the major proabortion victories. The Court struck down a local city ordinance requiring (1) last trimester abortions to be performed in a hospital (as opposed to a clinic or doctor's office), (2) minors under the age of 15 to have a parent's or court's permission for an abortion, (3) informed consent information designed to influence the woman's decision and irrelevant to the medical procedure (a "parade of horribles" to use one expression) to be provided to the patient, (4) a 24-hour waiting period to precede any abortion, and (5) humane disposal of fetal remains by the abortion provider. The court recognized that such requirements were more to discourage a person from freely choosing a constitutionally guaranteed procedure, rather than justifiably regulating the procedure.

In 1982 Ronald Reagan's election signaled a general turning point in our country. A more conservative element began to take over in legislative and judicial halls. By the time 1989 rolled around, the face of the Court had changed dramatically. It was this year that pro-life forces saw their first major victory in the Supreme Court. The case was *Webster v. Reproductive Health Services* and the court ruled on it on July 3, 1989. Missouri had passed a statute in 1986 that enacted several restrictions on abortions. The preamble of the statute read that the "life of each human being begins at conception."[7] Two of the restrictions were: (1) it outlawed abortions after 20 weeks and required physicians to test all women seeking abortions; (2) it forbade the use of government funds, employees, and properties to be used in performing or counseling for nontherapeutic abortions. The statute was challenged in district court and was struck down. The Supreme Court reversed the district court's ruling and reinstituted the statute. In doing so the Court rejected the earlier "trimester" model used in *Roe v. Wade* as ineffective. The legislative barrier of the "first two trimesters" was now lifted. Also the court ruled that the statement in the preamble concerning when life begins was a statement of belief having no legal force and therefore could remain.

Ronald Reagan's election signaled a turning point in judicial decisions.

On June 25, 1990, two cases were ruled on that were strong pro-life victories. In *Hodgson v. Minnesota* and *Ohio v. Akron Center for Reproductive Health* the court affirmed state statutes requiring minors to obtain either parental notification or court-appointed guardian notification in order to receive an abortion. Then on May 23, 1991, the court ruled in *Rust v. Sullivan* that the federal government could withhold funds provided to health care organizations under Title X of the Public Health Services Act if such organizations "counsel or encourage abortion as a method of family planning."[8] The Reagan administration had issued this "gag" order which was challenged in the Supreme Court. The court ruled that it was not unconstitutional, and therefore could stand. (Bill Clinton's first act as president was the removal of this order.)

Things were looking positive for the pro-life side and some were predicting that any day would see the overruling of *Roe v. Wade*. However, that day was not to come. In 1992 the Court made its ruling on *Casey v. Planned Parenthood of Western Pennsylvania*. In many ways it was a victory for the pro-life movement. It upheld four of the five sections of the Pennsylvania Abortion Control Act (1989) including: (1) requirement of minors to obtain consent of parent or court appointed guardian to get an abortion, (2) a required 24-hour waiting period between informed consent and the procedure, and (3) a requirement that "informed consent" of the patient include information concerning fetal development, effects of abortion on both the patient and the fetus, and alternative solutions. However, the Court struck down a portion of the law requiring women to notify husbands of their intent to obtain an abortion. They felt this placed an undue burden on the woman and invaded her right to privacy.

When *Casey* was announced, few felt they had won any victories. However, the greatest blow to the pro-life movement was that the Court made it clear that they had no intention of overturning *Roe v. Wade*. In the majority opinion authored by three of the more conservative justices — O'Conner, Souter, and Kennedy — they wrote:

> But when the court does act in this way, its decision requires an equally rare precedential force to counter the inevitable efforts to overturn it and thwart its implementation. Some of those efforts may be mere unprincipled emotional reactions; others may proceed from principles worthy of profound respect. But whatever the premises or opposition may be, only the most convincing justification under the accepted standards of precedent could suffice to demonstrate that a later decision overruling the first was anything but a surrender to political pressure, and an unjustified repudiation of the principle on which the Court staked its authority in the first instance. So to overrule under fire in the absence of the most compelling reasons to reexamine a watershed decision would subvert the Court's legitimacy beyond any serious question.[9]

The court made it clear thay had no intention of overturning Roe v. Wade.

Since *Casey* the Supreme Court has been unwilling to consider any other case which even hints toward challenging the fundamental ideas in *Roe v. Wade*. In the past seven years, pro-life advocates have concentrated on regulating abortion, mostly on the state level. Most of these have been regulations concerning minors needing parental notification, restrictions concerning state funds being used to finance nontherapeutic abortions, and restrictions concerning certain types of abortions such as late-term abortions and partial-birth abortions. While the congressional movement for a ban on partial-birth abortions has not, to date, been successful in getting beyond a presidential veto, 24 states have passed state statutes outlawing partial-birth abortions and several more have legislation pending. The National Abortion Rights Action League reports that in 1998 states enacted 62 new laws that are restrictive of abortions.[10]

However, even with the victories achieved by the pro-life movement, abortion on demand is still available in many parts of the country for any reason, including sex selection, birth control, pregnancies out of wedlock, and eugenic reasons (bone marrow transplants). The most recent available statistics[11] are: 1,210,000 abortions per year, which translates into about 3,300 abortions per day, or 1 abortion every 30 seconds.

The Moral Arguments for and against Abortion

We turn now to moral arguments concerning abortion. It is important to note that we are looking at *moral* arguments, not necessarily *legal* arguments here. It is possible for something to be morally wrong and not legally wrong, and the opposite is true. Also one has legal rights and, many argue, one also has moral rights and these may not always correlate. A prostitute in the state of Nevada may have a legal right to solicit business, but many would question whether she has a moral right to do so. It is important in going through these arguments to remember this distinction.

There are generally three positions taken on this issue. The proabortion position (also known as the pro-choice view) holds that it is always, or almost always, morally permissible for a women to have an abortion. The opposite view is the pro-life view (also known as the antiabortion view) which holds that it is always, or almost always, immoral for a woman to have an abortion. Finally there is a moderate view which attempts to be somewhere in the middle. This view holds that abortion is usually not morally permissible, but under certain circumstances can regretfully be permitted. Oftentimes moderates will argue that the personhood of the fetus simply cannot be determined for certain. They will hold that it is more likely not a **person** early in the pregnancy and more likely a person later in the pregnancy. Therefore earlier abortions are more justifiable than later ones. Actually there are several different moderate views, depending on the particular circumstances one has in mind. The more conservative moderate view would allow abortions when the life of the mother is in danger. A bit less conservative are those who allow abortions both for danger to the mother's life and if the conception was the result of rape or incest. Finally a liberal moderate position would allow the preceding exceptions and would also include the situation where the child suffers from extreme deformities, its life expectancy would be very short, or even more liberal, if it is not wanted. While these positions are clear in some respects, like most things they tend to blend into each other at the edges and it's not always easy to see small differences. We will look briefly at some of the main arguments for each of these positions and then concentrate on what seems to be the core issue, the personhood of the unborn.

Proabortion Arguments
There are many different proabortion arguments. Dr. Francis J. Beckwith lists at least 68 separate and distinct arguments in his excellent book *Politically Correct Death: Answering Arguments for Abortion Rights* (Baker, 1993). It is outside the scope of this volume to examine all the different possible proabortion arguments. I will instead concentrate on the main three types of proabortion arguments. Each type has a number of possible variables.

1. ***The Right to Privacy Argument.*** This argument states that everyone has an absolute right to privacy concerning what to do with their body. This moral argument is based on the principle of respect for autonomy which includes a basic right to keep things private and personal if one wants to do so. There is a point to this argument — most of us recognize that people do have a moral right to a private life. It would be morally wrong for me to walk into your house and start going

through your things. It would be an invasion of privacy. The question is how "absolute" that right is.

Most would argue that the right to privacy can be infringed in certain situations, for example to protect the welfare of other people. Most of us recognize that your right to privacy does not allow you to act in a manner that endangers the public welfare. You cannot drive down the road any way you choose at any speed you desire and claim right to privacy. You also cannot abuse your own children. If you were doing so, it would not be immoral for someone to step in and stop you from harming them, even though we recognize that the relationship between child and parent is normally a private affair. All of our child abuse laws are based on such concepts.

The fetus is not a part of the woman's body.

Pro-life proponents argue that the same situation is true in a pregnancy. The fetus is not a part of the woman's body — it is her child. The fetus is a genetically distinct separate individual person with its own gender, blood type, and identity. It is not like an arm or organ that a person is said to possess. It is an individual attached to the mother, but not part of her body. When a zygote attaches itself to the wall of the uterus around the eighth day of pregnancy, the mother's body immediately recognizes this as a foreign entity and begins an immunological attack on the embryo which only survives by its own built-in defense system. The woman's body recognizes that this is not a part of her, even though it is dependent on her for its life.

One person who has argued for abortion based on right to privacy is Judith Jarvis Thomson. Her 1971 essay "A Defense of Abortion" is easily the most influential and widely read article on abortion.[12] In that essay she uses the illustration of a famous violinist who is in need of a kidney in order to live. It is determined that you are the only person who is a match.

So you are kidnapped and forceably attached to this violinist so that he can share your kidneys. If you unplug yourself from him, you will kill him. Do you have an obligation to remain strapped to the violinist? After all, he is a person with a right to life who is depending on you to help him stay alive. Therefore don't you have an obligation to let him stay strapped to you? If you don't, then, by analogy, neither does a woman have an obligation to keep a fetus "strapped" to her.

There is a difference between actively killing someone and passively allowing someone to die.

A number of problems with Thomson's analogy can be presented, but I will only mention two. First, there is a major difference between the relationship between you and the violinist and a mother and her child. I may or may not have an obligation to the violinist, but we recognize that parents have *prima facie* obligations to care for their children and children have *prima facie* claims on their parents to be cared for. All of our child abuse and abandonment laws stem from this basic understanding of the family unit. If a parent had a three-year-old that needed serious medical attention, but decided she didn't have any obligations to help the child, most people would say there is something very defective in that parent's reasoning. Philosopher Stephen Schwartz comments: "The very thing that makes it plausible to say [as Thomson says] that the person in bed with the violinist has no duty to sustain him, namely that he is a stranger unnaturally hooked up to him, is precisely what is absent in the case of the mother and her child"[13] Second, there is a difference between actively killing someone and passively allowing someone to die. We will discuss this distinction in more detail in the next chapter, however it is important to note that unplugging oneself from the violinist is analogous to removing someone who is dying from life supporting mechanisms. Soon the kidney disease that is affecting the violinist will take over and he will die. But he is dying from the disease, not from your not being attached to him. However, the child is being actively killed in an abortion procedure. Therefore Thomson's illustration does not work and a right to privacy does not give one the right to kill one's own children.

2. *The Quality of Life Argument*. This argument basically holds that if a child is deformed or defective it should not be forced to suffer through "a life worse than death." This is argued on different levels: some argue on the basis of the child's suffering itself, others on the burden that such a child might place on the family. The amount of suffering is also a variable in different forms of this argument. Some are referring to severe deformities, or situations where a child would only live for a very short period, while others would place any deformity into the argument such as mild retardation or Down's Syndrome.

This kind of argument has several problems. First, if in fact the fetus is a person, then she has the same moral rights and we have the same obligations to her as to any other person. Most all agree that we certainly would not take the life of a deformed or defective child or adult purely because they are deformed.[14] No matter how badly we might feel for them, to do so would be the worst form of discrimination. This leads to the second problem with this argument. Any quality-of-life argument is going to depend heavily on subjective standards of what makes a life worth living. However, it is presumptuous to claim that certain lives just aren't worth living because they don't meet a certain standard. In fact, it is interesting to note that not one handicapped or disability organization has come out in favor of abortion of those who are deformed or defective. If the pro-abortionists were right in using this argument, one would expect to see large numbers of **suicides** of those who were suffering or disabled. While there have certainly been some, it has not been at all what one would expect if the general feelings of the disabled were as the pro-abortionists imagine. Third, there is a logical problem with arguing that no life is better than a life of suffering. It is basically arguing that nothing is better than something. However, there is no logical way you can argue this, because in order to compare two things they both have to exist and have properties to compare. "Nothing" does not exist and has no properties, so one cannot compare it to anything, even something bad, and say that it is better. Finally, even if this argument were to make sense, the vast majority of abortions that take place don't fit into this category, and therefore it cannot be used to justify abortion as a fundamental reproductive right.

> *If the fetus is a person, then whatever reason justifies our taking its life would be the same for any other adult person walking around.*

3. *The Nonperson Argument.* This argument says that the duty to do no harm applies only to persons. The unborn fetus, especially in the first and second trimester, has not attained the status of being a person. Therefore the duty to do no harm does not apply to the fetus. Again there is a good point behind this argument. Moral obligations are something that normally apply to persons. I do not have a moral obligation to my car, to my office, or to the computer I am writing on. If I were to take a hammer to the computer, I might regret it, but I have not wronged it. It seems that this argument, if right, may have a point. However, it is going to depend on what a person is and if we have good reason to believe that a fetus is one. Since we will examine that issue more closely below, we will leave this argument for now. This argument gets the credit of hitting the nail on the head — *this* is the main issue in the abortion debate. If the fetus is a person, then whatever reason justifies our taking its life would be the same as for any adult person walking around. There are many other proabortion arguments: dangers of an illegal abortion, poverty, the child will be unwanted and unloved, etc. However, all of these have no force if the fetus is a person.

Even the moderate's position concerning rape and incest fails if the fetus is a person. Should the life of an innocent person be taken for an action he did not commit? Would we be free to take the life of an adult person if he had been the result of rape or incest? While not denying the trauma and tragedy of such an incident as rape or incest, it is highly doubtful that killing the unborn will really resolve this issue or make it go away. The question of personhood is the single most important question in the abortion debate.

Pro-Life Arguments

Again there are many different types of appeals and arguments from the pro-life camp. Even though this book argues from the pro-life position, we must acknowledge that not all these arguments are good ones. For example, some pro-lifers have attempted to show that abortion is wrong by holding up pictures of aborted children and showing how much they "look" human or by showing how the fetus can feel pain at a certain stage. These arguments are misguided, and they give the wrong impression. The impression is given that if it looks human, or feels pain, then it is a human person. The problem is that the opposite impression, while not logically necessary, is also given: if it doesn't look human or feel pain, then it is not a human person. However for those of us who believe the unborn is a person from the moment of conception, what it looks like or what it feels is not the issue.

A number of good arguments are available for the pro-life position. Don Marquis provides an argument that is based on an analysis of why killing is wrong.[15] He argues that what makes killing wrong is that it robs a person of the activities, experiences and enjoyments that would have constituted one's future. These are intrinsic goods that are wrong to take away. Marquis's point is not that the fetus is necessarily a person, a question he believes can remain open for the present, but that the fetus does have the future of a person and therefore to abort it is to rob it of that future.

Another argument is provided by Harry J. Gensler who argues on the basis of consistency using a Golden Rule approach in a style reminiscent of Kant's categorical imperative.[16] He says that a consistent person will not have one moral position for others and an opposite position for himself. If people are going to be consistent, they must expect of themselves what they would expect of others. If I think it is normally wrong for someone to steal from me, then it is normally wrong for me to steal from someone else. Consistency demands that I hold both of these beliefs. Applying this to abortion, if I am consistent and think abortion is normally morally permissible, then I would have to consent to the idea of having been aborted myself in normal circumstances. Since most people would not consent to having been aborted, most people would have to agree that abortion is normally impermissible, if they are going to be consistent.

Both of these arguments have much to commend them, though they have some problems as well. In general, they don't go as far as they can. The strongest pro-life argument is the personhood argument, and it is that argument to which we now turn.

The Personhood Argument

The personhood argument holds that the fetus is a full human person from conception, and therefore the duty to do no harm applies to the fetus regardless of quality of life. Patrick Lee summarizes the argument well in a syllogism:

> Intentionally killing an innocent person always is morally wrong.
> Abortion is the intentional killing of an innocent person.
> Therefore, abortion is always morally wrong.[17]

In order to understand this argument fully we need to analyze two issues: What is a person, and when does one begin?

The Concept of Personhood

What is a person? In asking the question we need to make some distinctions in terminology. For the present we will separate the terms "human" and "person." Human can be an ambiguous term in that it can be used a couple of different ways. One way we can use it is in the sense of a "human organism."

This is a biological/genetic concept. By this term we are speaking of a member of the human species determined by their DNA and by a particular physicalistic way of functioning. However, "human" can also be used to speak of the entire "human being" which would be a combination of human organism and personhood. Because of this possible confusion, I will be using the term "person" or "human person" in my discussion below. The term "person" is a philosophical nonphysicalistic concept. One cannot determine personhood purely through scientific investigation. Also it is important to realize that not all persons are necessarily human, and therefore one cannot equate the two as identical. God and angels are nonhuman persons. It is possible that aliens from different worlds (if any exist) could be persons. A "human person" then is a species or type of the genus "person."

> ### *One cannot determine personhood purely through scientific investigation.*

What are the necessary and sufficient conditions for something to be a person? What we are looking for are those properties or qualities that a thing must have in order to be a person — they are essential for it to be a person. What might these properties be? A number of philosophers have attempted to list some of these. Joel Feinberg states the following:

> It is because people are conscious, have a sense of their personal identities; have plans, goals, and projects; experience emotions; are liable to pains, anxieties, and frustrations; can reason and bargain, and so on — it is because of these attributes that people have . . . a personal well-being of a sort we cannot ascribe to unconscious or nonrational beings.[18]

Philosopher Mary Ann Warren draws up a similar list:

> 1. Consciousness (of objects and events external and/or internal to the being), and in particular the capacity to feel pain

2. Reasoning (the *developed* capacity to solve new and relatively complex problems)

3. Self-motivated activity (activity which is relatively independent of either genetic or direct external control)

4. The capacity to communicate, by whatever means, messages of an indefinite variety of types, that is, not just with an indefinite number of possible contents, but on indefinitely many possible topics

5. The presence of a self-concept and self-awareness, either individual or racial, or both.[19]

Warren herself does not claim this list is exhaustive. However, she claims that a person who has *none* of these five could not be rightfully called a person. Other lists of the properties of personhood have been drawn up, but they will contain similar properties: Consciousness of the external world, self-consciousness, self-determination, rational capacities, emotional expressions, willful direction, and communicative/social abilities are almost universally found on most lists of properties essential to be a person.

However, the status of these properties is something that is very important in our understanding of what a person is. If you will note, the way they are listed by both Feinberg and Warren are, for the most part, in terms of *presently functioning*. In other words, their position is that a person is one who functions in a certain way. This might be called a "**functionalistic**" definition of personhood. According to both Feinberg and Warren, a fetus is not a person because it is not presently functioning like one and, at the present moment, cannot function like one. However, there is another way to think of these properties — not as presently functioning, but as having the potential or *capacity* to function in this manner.

If we think about it, there are many times that these properties are not functioning in what we consider to be normal human persons, such as when you are in a deep sleep, in a coma, or under sedation. Certainly at these times you are not conscious of the outside world or yourself, have no ability to make decisions that would be characterized as self-determined, you are not reasoning, emotionally expressing yourself, or communicating with anyone. Yet we would certainly not say that you are not a person at that point. Someone cannot kill you while you are asleep and claim that they didn't kill a person because you weren't presently functioning as one. Perhaps it is better to say that a person is one who has the capacities for functioning according to the above listed properties.

However, we can't stop there. Someone might argue, "OK, we obviously have the capacity to function that way, because we will soon wake up and begin to immediately function as a person. However, the unborn does not have that ability. Therefore, it still cannot be considered a person." First I am not sure what time has to do with it. The unborn, if allowed to live and naturally cared for, will someday function that way — it's just a matter of time. It is true that the capacity in a full grown adult is more immediate, but time should not be the determining issue concerning personhood. Second, there is something more important here. This immediate capacity to function as a person can only be present if something more basic is present.

There is something about a human person that gives him the capacity to function as a person.

There is something about a human person that gives him this immediate capacity to function as a person. It is something that seems to belong to him by nature of what he is — a human being. Some have simply called this our "human nature." Others refer to it as our essence or our soul. Stephen Schwartz calls it our **basic inherent capacity**."[20] Only humans seem to have this (at least in the present world). Cows will never function as persons, not because they don't have the immediate capacity to function, but because they don't have any kind of capacity by nature of the kind of thing they are. But humans are a kind of thing that has these capacities. We only have an *immediate* capacity to function as a person because we have a more basic *inherent* capacity to function as a person that is there by nature of what we are.

This brings out an important distinction — the distinction between *being* and *doing*. In order for a being to do something, it has to exist. Existence must always precede action. In relation to personhood, a person must already exist in order to function as one. It is not the functioning that *makes* one a person, she already *is* a person — that is why she is functioning that way. It is the *being* a person that grants one the capacity to *function* as a person. This is an extremely important distinction and one that we shall return to a number of times in this book.

With this in mind, how might we define "human person"? Philosopher J.P. Moreland defines a person this way: "A genus that takes being human as a species constituted by a fairly standard set of highest order capacities for mental states and for forming a body (in the case of human personhood)."[21] By "constituted by a fairly standard set of highest order capacities" I take Moreland to be saying that these capacities are there by nature of the kind of being a human person is. What might we list as the "fairly standard set" of capacities? The actual list is not necessarily important. There are certain capacities that most would agree on. I would say, at least minimalistically, four capacities are essential for a being to be a person: the capacity for rational reflection, emotional expression, willful direction, and to be morally conditioned. Certainly these are debatable, but I believe they sum up the essence of what a person is.

However, there is one more issue we need to discuss. There will be those who might say, "There are some in the world whom we would consider to be persons, but who do not have these capacities. For example, severely retarded people do not have the capacity for rational reflection or willful direction. Or people in a coma." I believe humans in these unfortunate states are still persons and have these capacities, they are just unable to access them to function properly. Philosopher Stephen Schwartz describes these situations as "latent capacities." A **latent capacity** is one that is present, but is inaccessible due to permanent or temporary damage, blockage, or underdevelopment. Schwartz writes:

> Even a very severely abnormal or handicapped human being has the basic inherent capacity to function as a person, which is a sign that he is a person. The abnormality represents a *hindrance* to the actual working of this capacity, to its manifestation in actual functioning. It does not imply the *absence* of this capacity, as in a nonperson.[22]

There are some whom we would consider to be persons, but who lack the capacities we use to define personhood.

This is why we recognize that it is a tragedy when someone is impaired or disabled either physically or mentally. We recognize that it is not the normal way they should be by nature of what they are. A table cannot think, communicate with others, make plans or perform actions. Yet we do not think that it is a tragedy that a table cannot do these things for tables are, by nature, not supposed to function this way. But human persons, by nature, are supposed to function in these ways. In admitting that something is wrong with a human in this state of affairs, we are admitting that he is a kind of creature who by nature should be otherwise.

We now have a pretty good idea of what a human person is. The question we wish to turn to next is when does one begin.

When Does Personhood Begin?

To begin with, it is important to realize what the question is asking and what it is not asking. The question is not "When does the human organism come into being?" Any medical scientist will tell you that the human organism is formed at the moment of conception. The zygote has its own genetic code and is considered a separate entity right from the start. What the question is asking is, when does it become a person? There are three general answers to this question: (1) we don't know, (2) at a decisive moment in the pregnancy, and (3) personhood gradually develops over the course of the entire pregnancy. These three possible answers should be examined in detail.

1. The Agnostic Theory

This theory says that no one can really know when personhood begins. It says the philosophers, scientists, theologians, and lawyers all disagree as to the beginning of personhood. No one has demonstrated anything with 100% certainty. Since no one can really know when personhood begins, they say, we should not entertain the question and the issue of personhood should not be a relevant one. Therefore, except for other possible ethical issues in a given situation (like informed consent, etc.), abortion is justifiable.

A number of problems with this theory present themselves. First, there are a couple of logical problems with this view. In the first place, if it is really true that "no one knows" when personhood begins, then what is to stop someone from killing a two-year-old because he believed that personhood didn't occur until three? This is an example of a logical fallacy called the argument of the beard. It got its name by noting that, because we can't pinpoint exactly when stubble ends and a beard begins, we can't say we know if something really is a beard or not. However, just because we may not be able to know the exact moment personhood might occur (a position I am not granting), doesn't mean we can't know anything at all. Most people certainly know a two-year-old is a person and would condemn anyone for murdering one. Therefore personhood must go back farther than that. If we examine the properties that make a two-year-old a person, we may be able to understand if the fetus is one. There is a second logical problem with saying we "can't know" when personhood begins — it is making a knowledgeable claim about something it says no one can know. In other words, how does the agnostic know something about the beginning of personhood (that we don't know when it begins), if in fact nobody can know about the beginning of personhood? The claim is self-defeating.

Second, if we truly grant that we can't know if the fetus is a person, that does not automatically lead one to justify abortion. In fact, it should lead to the opposite action. For, if we can't or don't really know, then we must acknowledge the real possibility that in fact it *could* be a person. If it is possible that it could be a person, then the benefit of the doubt goes to that possibility. To act any other way would be considered negligent homicide. If I am out hunting with friends and we divide up and I hear a rustling in the bushes, if I take aim and fire without first determining if it is a deer or a friend, I am acting in a negligent manner. If I shoot, and it turns out to be a friend who dies as a result of my shooting him, then I am guilty of negligent homicide. Even if it is *not* my friend, I am still guilty of criminal negligence for it could have been he. The same charge could be laid at the feet of the agnostic.

> *If we don't know whether the fetus is a person, we must acknowledge that it could be.*

A third problem with this view is that it is guilty of making the assumption that killing a human organism that is not a person is morally justifiable. Now, there are those who hold that such a separation cannot be. Assuming for the sake of argument that these two aspects can be separated, the assumption that killing a human organism is morally justifiable, just not killing a human person, has not been defended. It is certainly possible that a human organism may be the kind of thing that one just can't treat any way one wants. After all, eagle eggs have laws that protect them, so why not human organisms? Many would argue that to torture an animal to death is morally wrong, and yet that is not a person. Finally some, like Don Marquis above, would argue that we should not kill human organisms because, even if they are not currently persons, they have a future as human persons.

A fourth problem with this view is that by allowing abortion on demand, agnostics have for all practical purposes already decided when a human organism becomes a human person: sometime after birth. This is when the agnostic grants the person its rights not to be harmed or killed and when we have duties toward it. However, there is no real difference in the actual being itself one hour before birth or one hour after it. Some agnostics will say that they feel certain that it is probably a person sometime earlier than birth, they are just not sure when that might be. However, just like with the event of birth, if pressed they will be forced to select an event in pregnancy at which they will draw the line. This leads to our next theory: decisive moment theories.

2. Decisive Moment Theories

The **decisive moment** theories say that there is a decisive moment in the pregnancy when the person comes into existence. Eight possible decisive moments can be pointed to as possible events when the person could come into existence.

a. *Conception*. This has been the traditional view of the beginning of personhood and there are good reasons to hold this view. First, there is a radical break that occurs here that does not occur any other time in the pregnancy. In conception two things (sperm and egg) become one thing, a zygote. A whole new entity that did not previously exist, comes into existence and two other entities, sperm and egg, cease to exist. Some might reply, "But the egg still exists, it has just been fertilized." However, that is to miss the point. It is not a "fertilized egg," for the moment it became fertilized it ceased being an egg. Not only is this true on the conceptual level, but also on the biological level. Schwartz explains:

> The expression *fertilized egg* (or ovum) is also scientifically wrong. The new human being is no more the egg fertilized than he is the sperm fertilized, or modified. He is as little the one as the other, but a new being. The ovum is merely bigger than the sperm, hence the tendency to speak of it as a fertilized egg, but each contributes exactly one half to the genetic makeup of the new person. And in the process, each ceases to be.[23]

The fact that there is such a radical break at this point where a new being comes into existence provides, in the absence of defeaters, strong *prima facie* evidence that personhood begins here as well.

Second, this new being is a completely separate individual with its own genetic code, needing only food, water, shelter and oxygen in order to develop, grow and continue its existence. It is not a "part" of the mother's body and nothing substantively new will ever be added to it that will change it in any dramatic way.

The fetus is a completely separate individual with its own genetic code.

Third, metaphysically speaking, this new being is a particular kind of *being* with a nature and it is in the process of *becoming* in accordance with that nature. It is not a "becoming" who is striving toward "being." It is not a potential human person, but a human person with potential limited only by its nature. It is *essentially* a human person; that is why it develops as a person instead of as something else. Personhood is there from the beginning; that is why it will develop as a person. Sunflower seeds develop as sunflowers, watermelon seeds develop as watermelons, human persons develop as persons. If personhood is not there from the beginning, at least in latent form, where did it come from? Any other theory is going to have to answer that question.

Fourth, this new being is the product of human parents. Whatever is the sexual product of members of a species is itself an individual member of that species. Since the species "human" includes, by nature, the quality of personhood, a member of that species will have that quality. In fact, a subcommittee of the Senate Judiciary Committee made this comment in its report after listening to witnesses testify concerning the 1981 Human Life Bill, "No witness [who testified before the subcommittee] raised any evidence to refute the biological fact that from the moment of conception there exists a distinct individual being who is alive and is of the human species. No witness challenged the scientific consensus that unborn children are 'human beings' in so far that the term is used to mean living beings of the human species."[24]

Fifth, the new person conceived has continuity through time. The same person which began at conception as a zygote will continue through birth, childhood, adolescence, and adulthood as the essentially same person. There is no other radical break. You did not come *from* a zygote, you *were* a zygote, just like you did not come from an adolescent, you were an adolescent. No stage of our development, inside or outside of the womb imparts us with our personhood. That is why it is proper to say "When I was conceived . . . ." The only place to draw the line is conception.

Sixth, personhood must begin at conception by process of elimination. No other event in the development of the fetus can account for when personhood begins. As we shall see, all other events suffer from a lack of explanatory power on this question.

No other event than conception can account for when personhood begins.

b. *Implantation.* Implantation occurs 6-8 days after conception. This occurs after the new zygote moves down through the fallopian tube where conception occurred and implants itself on the uterine wall. Some believe that personhood cannot occur before this event for a number of reasons. Bernard Nathanson argues for this because this is the time when the zygote establishes its presence by "transmitting signals" (hormones) and "interfacing" with the human community.[25] Communication with the outside world is essential for personhood. There are two problems with this view. First, there is a difference between *being* and *knowledge of being*. It is possible for something to exist and for us to have no knowledge of its existence. In fact, there probably exist many things in the universe of which no one is aware. That does not mean they do not exist. The essence of what a thing is does not depend on others' awareness of the thing's existence. Second, what about conceptions that occur *in vitro*? Any child conceived this way has "communicated its presence" before implantation.

Another reason some argue for implantation as recognition of personhood is that some products of conception are not human beings at all. Therefore, they reason, being conceived is not what makes you human, and one is wrong to argue that life begins at conception. What they are referring to are certain things like hydatiform moles (a degenerated placenta), choriocarcinoma (conception cancer), or a blighted ovum (placenta lacking an embryonic plate). The problem with this argument is that it confuses necessary and sufficient conditions of being human. Just because human persons begin at conception doesn't imply that all things that begin at conception are human. This is the fallacy of illicit conversion. It is saying that **A**: "All human persons are things that begin at conception" implies **B**: "All things that begin at conception are human persons." But since **B** is not true, proven by the examples given above, then **A** must not be true either. However, that is like saying that "All apples are fruit" implies "All fruit are apples" which obviously does not follow.

Some argue that implantation must be where personhood begins because 30% of all conceptions die before implantation. "Yet," they argue, "we don't treat these as humans. We don't try to save them or give them funerals." However, it doesn't follow logically that the new being conceived is not fully human just because it's not treated as such. If we treated a fully grown adult like this, it would not mean he is not a person. Unfortunately in our history we have not always treated people of different races as persons. In fact in the Dred Scott decision (1857) an African-American slave was declared only three-fifths a person. That didn't mean he wasn't a full person.

In the Dred Scott decision an African-American slave was declared only three-fifths a person.

The most formidable argument for implantation is the argument from segmentation or "twinning." This occurs before implantation. This argument says that a human person is essentially one absolute individual being. "Persons" cannot be split in two. Since the conceptus can be split in two, it must not be a person. There are a number of replies to this objection. First, every being conceived is still a genetically unique individual, distinct from her/his parent. Just because twins came from one conceptus, it does not logically follow that the conceptus is not fully human and a member of the human species having, by nature, personhood. It just happens in the case of twins that the genetic code each possesses is identical to the other. This is also true after birth, but we wouldn't kill them then either. Second, there is no logical contradiction in having two persons existing in one physical conceptus. From Siamese twins we know that two individuals can be joined together and share the same body parts, such as the heart or even the head, and yet we recognize that they are separate persons and always have been. The two newly conceived persons are joined in the same manner, just more closely. What we are arguing is that all human conceptions contain at least one person, but not necessarily only one. Finally, Patrick Lee comments:

> When a person is defined as a certain type of *individual*, the word means *logically* undivided as opposed to a universal or class, where the property or nature is divided among many. The division of the embryo shows only that he or she is *physically* divisible. . . The fact is that all of us are *physically* divisible, but that does nothing to call into question our present individuality in the relevant sense.[26]

c. *Brain Development.* About 15 days after conception the "primitive streak" appears that will develop into the brain and nervous system. By the 20th day the foundation for the brain and spinal cord is established and by the 33rd day the cerebral cortex is formed. Some argue that since a human being is considered dead at brain death, the person no longer exists in the body at this time, therefore it seems logical that when the brain begins to function, that is when personhood starts. They argue that you cannot have a person without a brain because there is no capacity for consciousness. There may be good reasons for arguing that with no brain, there is no capacity for those properties which we identified earlier as distinctive of what a person is. Certainly there is normally a strong relationship between brain states and the mental states necessary for a person to function. However, I don't think this argument works for a couple of reasons. First, the argument assumes a symmetry exists between brain-death and brain-life. If the "person" is gone at brain death, then he must not be there until the brain is alive. As much as this symmetry *seems* to exist, there is no *a priori* reason to assume it really exists. There is no evidence for it; it is just our tendency to be symmetrical.

In fact, there is a big difference between "brain death" and "no brain yet." A dead person has lost the natural inherent capacity to live. The brain does not have the capacity to work because it has irreversibly ceased — it is dead. However, the unborn has not lost the natural inherent capacity to live. The capacity is there from conception and it is still living. Therefore, the absence of brain activity is not necessarily the same as the death of the brain.

> ### *There is a big difference between "brain death" and "no brain yet."*

Second, the statement that the unborn has "no capacity for consciousness without a brain" is somewhat ambiguous. If one is speaking of immediate capacity, then the statement is true. But the unborn does possess the essential structure for this capacity, so he does have the capacity in a latent form. Where would it come from if he didn't already have it? Nothing substantial is added to the fetus after conception that would explain where the brain comes from. Again, because he cannot function like a person, doesn't mean he is not one. One can argue that the brain has not fully developed in an infant, yet most would recognize that an infant is a person.

d. *The Appearance of Humanness.* Around 8-10 weeks the fetus begins to take on more and more of the appearance of being human. Facial features are apparent, hands and feet are almost fully formed, sex organs can be seen. There are those who argue that it is at this time that we begin to treat the unborn as a person. This argument is often subtly offered. Some will point to a picture or drawing of a zygote and say "How can you call *that* a person?" Pro-lifers will parade around pictures of aborted fetuses and proclaim, "See, you're killing little children!" However, both of these approaches to personhood are wrong. First, appearance is neither a sufficient nor a necessary condition to being a human person. One can have things appear as human persons which are not, such as manikins or robots like Data in the series *Star Trek: The Next Generation*, and one can be a human person without appearing as one: extremely deformed persons, badly burned victims, victims of massive amputations. Second, this objection assumes that personhood presupposes a certain form. However our outward human form changes considerably throughout our life from childhood, through adolescence and adulthood, to our elderly years. If appearance depends on a certain form, then at what point are we a person? Finally, this is prejudice and bigotry. The poor treatment of African-Americans in this country was, and unfortunately often still is, because they "look different."

e. *The Attainment of Sentience.* Somewhere between 8-13 weeks the unborn will begin to experience physical sensations such as pain. This is called **sentience**. Some argue that this is when the unborn should be treated as a person. This is based on the idea that a being that can feel pain has interests, and anything that has interests can be harmed. We have an obligation not to harm beings that can have interests, i.e., persons.[27] Pro-lifers have also used this argument in films like *The Silent Scream* where they show a baby feeling pain. Like the above argument based on appearance, while these have dramatic value, the problem again is that sentience is neither a sufficient nor necessary criterion for personhood. First, this view confuses **harm** with **hurt** and the experience of harm with the reality of harm. Hurt implies an awareness of pain; harm is the obstruction or prevention of the legitimate interests of one party by the invasive actions of another party. You can harm someone without ever hurting them. For example, if you tell me something in confidence and I tell your boss so you don't get a promotion, I've harmed you even if you don't know and never know you were up for a promotion and didn't get it. Hurt occurs when one experiences harm, but harm doesn't need to be experienced to really exist. If the fetus already is a person, you are harming it by aborting it, whether it ever feels it or not. Second, if sentience is **the** criterion for personhood, then anytime we are not sentient, we are not persons. That would include being in a deep sleep, comatose, unconscious, or under general anesthesia. Yet most would acknowledge that you are still a person even in these states. In fact, the unity between two sentient states implies the underlying person still exists even though he or she is not sentient at the moment. When you wake up, you are still the same person you were when you went to sleep. Therefore there must be more to being a person then sentience.

Harm doesn't need to be experienced to exist.

f. *Quickening.* Quickening is an old term to describe the first time movement of the unborn is felt by the mother, usually between 16-17 weeks. This is an ancient theory before modern medicine. It was thought that this is when the soul entered the body and therefore, marked the beginning of personhood. However, this is an example of a factual problem, not a moral problem. Those ancient and medieval scholars who condemned any abortion after quickening would surely do so today from conception. Again, knowing a person is there and a person being there are two different things that are unrelated. It is confusing epistemology with metaphysics.

g. *Viability*. Viability is the term used to describe when the baby can live outside of the womb. Today it is thought to be somewhere between 20-24 weeks, though this time frame is always getting pushed back further and further. The argument based on viability says that prior to this time the unborn is totally dependent on the special environment of the womb. The unborn then is not a completely independent human life and hence not fully human. This was the view suggested by the majority opinion in the *Roe v. Wade* case. However, there are problems with this argument. First, viability has nothing to do with transforming the nature of the fetus from nonperson to person. It is more of a comment on our medical technology, than on personhood. Second, viability changes with medical progress. The time of viability cannot be determined precisely. What was not a person in 1973 at 22 weeks is now accepted as a person in the 1990s. This seems to be an arbitrary designator of what is a person. Third, each one of us can be nonviable in relation to the outside environment. For example, without a special means or apparatus on the moon, underwater, or at the North Pole, we would not be able to survive in the outside environment. It doesn't make us less of a person just because we are dependent upon some special means for our survival. Finally, as Francis J. Beckwith points out, Justice Blackmun's argument in Roe v. Wade based on viability is circular.[28] Blackmun claims that the state only has an interest in protecting fetal life when it can live outside the womb. Why? Because prior to living outside the womb the fetus has no interests or rights. In other words, he is assuming (that the fetus has no rights) what he is trying to prove (that the fetus has no rights). However, he has provided no *independent* evidence for his conclusion that the fetus has no rights. It's like arguing that the Los Angeles *Dodgers* are the best team in baseball because no one is better.[29]

What was not a person in 1973 at 22 weeks is now accepted as a person in the 1990s.

h. *Birth*. In general, 40 weeks after conception a mother will give birth to a child. Some argue that since our society calculates the beginning of one's existence from birth (i.e., how old you are) and since it is only after birth that one is named and accepted into a family, then the child is not fully human until after birth. However, social customs and conventions have nothing to do with someone being a person. One is not less a person if unnamed, abandoned, or no one knows his or her birthday. A dog can be treated like a human (named, accepted into the family, celebrate its birthday) but that doesn't make it human. Also, there is no essential difference of an unborn child the day before birth and the day after birth. Its nature has not changed in any way. It is just a matter of location.

The decisive moment that has the best evidence going for it, and the most explanatory power is conception. The other theories have too many problems and offer no explanation for the origin of personhood. Therefore I believe that the person begins at conception. However, there is one other possibility that is fairly popular today. It is to that position we now turn.

Gradualism is the view that says there is no one specific moment when personhood begins. Instead it is a gradual change that occurs over the entire pregnancy. In the beginning, at conception, there is no person and by the end, at birth, there is a person. There is no one decisive moment between conception and birth, personhood slowly develops as the fetus develops. Some, like Judith Jarvis Thomson have used the acorn as an example: it gradually develops into an oak tree.[30] It certainly isn't an oak tree to begin with, but it is one at the end. Most gradualists would hold then, that the unborn gains moral rights, including the right to life, as it develops. A zygote has less rights than a fetus who, in turn, has less rights than a newborn. Therefore, earlier abortions are more easily justified than later abortions.

3. Gradualism

There are two main reasons why gradualists hold this view. First, they argue that it is simply impossible to draw a line for when personhood begins. We just don't know where to do it. It is better to abandon all decisive moment theories than to go on pretending we can know something that is just impossible to know. Second, the unborn close to birth seems very much like the rest of us, where the zygote simply doesn't. Philippa Foot, for example, expresses this view well when she says, ". . . as we go back in the life of the foetus we are more and more reluctant to say that this is a human being and must be treated as such"[31]

However there are some serious problems with the gradualist position. First, at best the theory is a hypothesis. There is absolutely no evidence to support it. It may "seem" that a zygote is very different from a baby, and one may be "reluctant" to call a zygote a person, however this is hardly evidence to support the view. Any evidence that could be offered would need to be very strong because it would have to overcome some tremendous difficulties as we will see below. Therefore it has a low degree of probability of being true.

Second, though there may be the gradual *development* of a person (physical, social, etc.), it is impossible to have the gradual process of *being* a person. There are only two possible concepts when it comes to existence: being and nothing. Things either exist or they don't. There is no such concept of something partially existing and partially not existing, or of something "becoming" into existence. What *exists* may develop, but there is no such thing as something "developing into existence." This is why you can trace your life back — adolescence, childhood, babyhood, fetus, embryo, zygote — *you* have developed, but you have always been you. The zygote was not you partly existing and you partly not existing. Development concerns functioning as a person, not being a person. Thomson's illustration actually supports this. An acorn has the basic inherent capacity to develop as an oak tree, that is why it develops as one. In the same manner the zygote has the basic inherent capacity to develop as a person, that is why it develops as one.

Third, if **gradualism** were true, the gradualist would have to hold to the awkward idea of beings like "half person/half nonperson." At the beginning there is no person and at the end there is a full person. Therefore there must have been a half-way point where there was a half-person, but what kind of person is a "half-person"? Person is a simple, undivided being.

Fourth, the gradualist ends up adopting an "assembly-line" picture of a person coming into being. For example, think of a car on an assembly line slowly coming into being as more parts are added to it. Gradualists apply this picture to the unborn in the womb. However it is a false analogy. Cars are artifacts that are created by adding several parts together; they are the sum of their parts. Persons are "natural kinds" and are living organisms. They are not the "sum of parts" because personhood is a "simple" idea — it has no parts and is not able to be divided up into parts.

Have we fully developed as persons at birth?

Finally, why does the gradualist stop at birth? Have we fully developed as persons at birth? Psychologists will tell you not even half-way psychologically. If you take gradualism to its logical conclusion, then the gradualist must affirm the absurd position that a baby is less a person than a two-year-old, and a two-year-old is less a person than a ten-year-old, and so on. Since the gradualist correlates the wrongness of killing a being with its development as a person, then it is less wrong to kill a two-year-old than a ten-year-old, and less to kill a ten-year-old than an adult. What the gradualist wants to do is limit this gradual development to pregnancy alone. However, that is inconsistent and contradictory. He says we can't draw a line, but that is what he is doing. If gradualism is true, then you can't draw a line to end development any more then you can draw a line to when a person begins, inside or outside the mother.

4. Conclusion

There is a point when personhood occurs — at the moment of conception. All other theories fail to provide an account for any other time personhood could come into existence; the agnostic and gradualist run into problems of inconsistency

and incoherence. Three continuums give evidence for personhood from conception to death: (1) The Continuum of
Identity: Because of our basic inherent capacity we keep the
same identity through time. The same person who was conceived and was a zygote is the same "self" that will be an
adult; (2) The Continuum of Essential Structure: the essential
structure for the basic inherent capacity to function as a
person is present at the moment of conception and remains in
various forms until death; and (3) The Continuum of Capacities: The basic inherent capacity is the basis for all the other
capacities needed in order to function as a person. I have present capacities to function as a person: reason, moral reflection, etc. But these are all based on the basic capacity I have
had from conception. There is no such thing as a "potential
person" just "the potential to function as a person." We may
not be able to achieve a satisfactory list of the properties of
personhood. But whatever it is, it appears to be in humans
from conception. At least the basic inherent capacity is.

There are only four possibilities.

We will conclude by noting what Christian philosopher
Peter Kreeft has written.[32] He writes that either a fetus is a
person or not and either we know it or not. Therefore there
are only four possibilities: (1) It is not a person and we know
it. If this were true, then abortion would be permissible. But
no one has been able to prove with any certainty that a fetus
is not a person and the preponderance of evidence points to
the opposite conclusion. (2) It is a person and we know it. If
this is true, then abortion is murder. (3) It is a person and we
don't know it. Then we are guilty of manslaughter. For we
have enough evidence to acknowledge it at least could be a
person (even the gradualist and agnostic admit that) and
therefore should have taken care not to have killed it. (4) It is
not a person and we don't know it. Then abortion is criminal
negligence. For again, even if it is not a person, we have

strong enough evidence to acknowledge it *could* be a person. Although we would not actually be killing a person under this option, we are acting in a criminally negligent manner. In short abortion never comes off under any of these options as the right action to take, and these are the only options.

What does Scripture say about abortion? Actually, it may surprise some to find that it doesn't say anything specific about abortion at all. Many pro-abortionists take this as tacit permission for abortion. However, it would be wrong to take that approach. If that was the correct method of handling Scripture, then one could argue that pedophilia is permissible because Scripture does not specifically address that issue. However, we might ask why Scripture does not address the issue. Part of it may stem from the fact that the very idea of abortion was contrary to the ancient Jewish view of having children. Children were seen as a blessing. In fact, for a woman to be barren was often interpreted as a curse from God and something to be lamented about. Roland de Vaux, who wrote the classic *Ancient Israel: Social and Religious Institutions* writes:

Scripture and Abortion

> In ancient Israel, to have many children was a coveted honor, and the wedding guests often expressed the wish that the couple would be blessed with a large family. . . . Sterility, on the other hand, was considered a trial (Gn 16:2; 30:2, Is 1:5) or a chastisement from God (Gn 20:18) or a disgrace from which Sarah, Rachel, and Leah all tried to clear themselves by adopting the child which their maids bore to their husbands (Gn 16:2; 30:3,9).[33]

Therefore, it should not be surprising that we find nothing in Scripture specifically addressing the abortion issue.

We find nothing in Scripture specifically addressing the abortion issue, but we do find comments on killing innocent persons.

However, we do find scriptural comments on killing innocent persons. The most obvious place is the fifth commandment, "You shall not murder" (Exod 20:13, NASB). What is it about murder that makes it so wrong? A number of answers have been raised. Murder robs society of someone of value to it or murder robs the murdered victim of a future are just two answers that have been proposed. However the scriptural answer has nothing to do with society and, surprisingly, nothing to do with the murdered person. Murder is something you do to God. It is an affront on his image. We see this in Genesis 9:6: "Whoever sheds man's blood, by man his blood shall be shed, *For in the image of God He made man*" (NASB, emphasis mine). The fact that man is made in the image of God places him in a very unique status in comparison to all else that has been created. There are no other restrictions as to the killing of other animals in any general sense. However, because of this privileged position, man may not be killed by any other man — to do so is to desecrate the image of God. There has been much speculation of what this image actually is. I believe, without going into details, the image is found in man's personhood. This is what separates man from all other creatures. As persons we are image-of-God bearers and we are obligated to respect that image.

Does Scripture give us an idea of when personhood, i.e., image of God, occurs? Again it doesn't make any specific comment. Any time Scripture talks about humans it always treats them as persons. There is no separation in Scripture between "human person" and "nonhuman person." However, perhaps we can approach the question differently. Christian philosopher Scott Rae suggests that the best approach is ". . . by equating the unborn child in the womb with a child or adult out of the womb."[34] He suggests the following argument:

1. God attributes the same characteristics to the unborn as to an adult [or child].
2. Therefore God considers the unborn a person.
3. Abortion is killing an innocent person.
4. Killing innocent persons violates the fifth commandment (Ex. 20:13).[35]

What are some characteristics of persons that God attributes to the unborn? First, the same language is used for the unborn (Luke 1:41,44) as is used for a child or baby who is already born (Luke 2:12,16). Second, the same punishments are meted out for the injury or killing of the unborn (Exod 21:22-25) as for killing or injuring an adult (Lev 24:19-20). Third, God claims to have knowledge of the unborn in a personal way using personal pronouns (Jer 1:5; Ps 139:15-16) as he uses of other persons. Fourth, God calls the unborn to their vocation (Isa 49:1) in the same way he calls other persons (Amos 7:14-15).

Along with the characteristics listed above, Scripture draws a continuity between conception and birth in personal terms. Genesis 4:1 tells us of the first birth: "Now the man had relations with his wife Eve, and she conceived and gave birth to Cain, and she said, 'I have gotten a manchild with *the help of* the LORD'"(NASB). There is a continuity of personhood from the conception of Cain to the Birth of Cain. Job 3:3 also draws the same continuity. Job is lamenting his situation and says, "Let the day perish on which I was to be born, And the night *which* said, 'A boy is conceived'"(NASB). Hebrew parallelism joins together the 'I' who was born with the 'boy' who was conceived. They are the same person.

Some pro-abortionists have pointed to Exodus 21:22-25 as implying that the fetus is not a full person:

> And *if* men struggle with each other and strike a woman with child so that she has a miscarriage, yet there is no *further* injury, he shall surely be fined as the woman's husband may demand of him; and he shall pay as the judges *decide*. But if there is *any further* injury, then you shall appoint *as a penalty* life for life, eye for eye, tooth for tooth, hand for hand, foot for foot, burn for burn, wound for wound, bruise for bruise (NASB).

Some pro-abortionists point out that the penalty for causing a miscarriage is less than the penalty for taking a life and that therefore the value of the fetus is less than a person. The problem with this interpretation is based on an unfortunate translation of this text in versions such as the New American

Standard Bible (normally a good version, but not here). The Hebrew word translated "miscarriage," *yahtzah*, in the above text literally means to "come forth" and is the standard term for giving birth. Since she was struck by one or more men, she gives birth prematurely. However, there is nothing in this passage that even implies it is a miscarriage. There is another Hebrew word for miscarriage, *shakol*, and that term is not in use here. Another problem with this translation is the insertion of the word "further" before "injury." In the NASB whenever a word is in italics, it is to inform the reader that this is an interpretive insertion and not in the original. If one removes the word "further" and translates "miscarriage" to "gives birth" the original meaning becomes clear: If two men are fighting and they strike a pregnant woman so that she gives birth, but there is no injury, then they only have to pay the husband a fine (to compensate for a premature birth). However, if there is injury then they must pay equal to the injury. And the penalty given here is exactly as that given in Leviticus 24 for injury to an adult: eye for an eye, tooth for a tooth, life for life. This passage supports the personhood of the unborn by stipulating the same penalty.

> *There is a Hebrew word for miscarriage, which is not used in Exodus 21:22.*

It seems clear from what we have seen that Scripture would support the personhood of the unborn. This is not necessarily presenting an open and shut case, but the evidence would certainly seem to lie on the pro-life side.

Conclusion   In looking at the personhood argument and considering what Scripture seems to teach, Christians have a good reason to believe that the unborn is a person from conception on. The final question is "Where do we go from here?" There are two basic responses a Christian can take. One response is to withdraw into one's own community and let the non-Christian world go its own way. The other response is to be actively involved in the abortion issue. This second response is called activism, and in the opinion of this author it is the preferable response. Christians should have a voice in the public square, sharing what they believe to be true. In fact, if they really believe it is true, they have an obligation to share it with others. However there are two kinds of activists: hard activists and soft activists. The hard activist will use any means to achieve his purpose. He will work both inside and outside the law if necessary. This is surely an incorrect response. Acts of violence against any other person in the name of "pro-life" are deplorable and self-contradictory. In a democratic pluralistic society we should, as much as we can, respect laws that are arrived at in a fair and equitable manner. However, soft activism should be encouraged. Soft activism is working within the laws and in respect of others by reasoning with individuals and encouraging legislative activity to change laws one believes are bad laws. The laws allowing abortion in this country certainly fall under the category of "bad laws." We should actively and respectfully attempt to change those laws. We have good reasons to support our view; we need to aggressively and respectfully share those reasons.

ENDNOTES

[1]Details concerning Norma McCorvey's story were gathered primarily from Michelle Green, "The Woman behind Roe v. Wade," *People Magazine* (May 22, 1989). It is interesting to note that in 1995 Norma announced that she had become a Christian and repudiated the court decision that she was responsible for. She worked with Operation Rescue for two years before beginning her own ministry in 1997, "Roe No More Ministry." She currently resides in Dallas, Texas.

[2]Some may question my selection of terms, so a comment is in order. I have decided to use the term "proabortion" instead of the more popular "pro-choice" because I believe it more accurately reflects their position on this debate. Despite the rhetoric, no one is questioning any person's "right to choose." A person has a right to choose anything they want. I have a right to choose to steal if I want (and am willing to accept the consequences of that choice). The question is not my right to choose, but whether that choice is morally appropriate. I believe the debate centers around the moral appropriateness of abortion and have chosen the term "proabortion" because those who hold that view believe abortion is, at least sometimes, morally appropriate. I have retained the term pro-life because I believe that is the focus of

those from that position. They believe abortion is morally inappropriate precisely because we are talking about killing a living person. The issue for them is the "life" of the person. If it wasn't a living person, they would not have a problem with abortion. Therefore their position is truly "pro-life."

[3]Doe v. Bolton, 410 U.S. 179 (1973).

[4]Ibid.

[5]U.S. Senate, Committee on the Judiciary, *Report on Human Life Bill*, S. 158, 1981, 5.

[6]I may need to clarify the difference between a **negative right** and a **positive right**. A negative right is also called a "right of noninterference." In a sense, it is a right to be left alone. These are also called liberty rights. It means you have certain rights to do things and, because of those rights, others are not allowed to interfere with your doing those things. For example, the right to worship in the manner you choose, means that others cannot interfere with how you worship. By far the majority of our constitutional rights are negative rights. A positive right means that you have the right for something to be given to you. Rather than leaving you alone, others must actively provide something to you. As an example, our welfare system is based on the premise that everybody has basic rights to housing, a decent meal, etc. Therefore the government has an obligation to provide these items to those who cannot afford them. Positive rights are more controversial than negative rights and usually harder to justify.

[7]*Webster v. Reproductive Health Services*, No. 88-605.

[8]*Rust v. Sullivan*, 500 U.S. 173 (1991).

[9]*Casey v. Planned Parenthood*, Nos. 91-744 and 91-902, V.

[10]Claudine Chamberlain, "Abortion Rights Reversal," ABCNews.com, Jan. 14, 1999.

[11]US Department of Health and Human Services, abortion statistics for 1995.

[12]Judith Jarvis Thomson, "A Defense of Abortion" (1971), reprinted in *The Abortion Controversy: A Reader*, ed. by Louis P. Pojman and Francis J. Beckwith (Boston: Jones and Bartlett, 1994), pp. 131-146.

[13]Stephen Schwartz, *The Moral Question of Abortion* (Chicago: Loyola University Press, 1990), p. 118.

[14]I am speaking of a person who has not requested that we take such action. Concerning those who make such requests, see chapter 4.

[15]Don Marquis, "Why Abortion is Immoral"(1989), in Pojman and Beckwith, *The Abortion Controversy*, pp. 320-338.

[16]Harry J. Gensler, "The Golden Rule Argument against Abortion"(1986), in Pojman and Beckwith, *The Abortion Controversy*, pp. 305-319.

[17]Patrick Lee, *Abortion and Unborn Human Life* (Washington, DC: Catholic University of America Press, 1996), p. 1.

[18]Joel Feinberg, "Abortion," in *Matters of Life and Death: New Introductory Essays in Moral Philosophy*, ed. by Tom Reagan (New York: Random House, 1986), pp. 256-293.

[19]Mary Ann Warren, "On the Moral and Legal Status of Abortion," *The Monist*, 57:1 (January, 1973): 43-61.

[20]Schwartz, *Moral Question*, p. 91, emphasis mine.

[21]J.P. Moreland, personal correspondence, December 16, 1998.

[22]Schwartz, *Moral Question*, p. 97, emphasis mine.

[23]Ibid., p. 70.

[24]Report of Subcommittee on Separation of Powers to Committee on the Judiciary, Human Life Bill — S.158, 97th Congress, 1981. Cited in Beckwith, *Politically Correct Death: Answering Arguments for Abortion Rights* (Grand Rapids: Baker, 1993), p. 43.

[25]Bernard Nathanson and Richard N. Ostling. *Aborting America* (Garden City, NY: Doubleday, 1979), p. 216.

[26]Lee, *Abortion*, p. 91.

[27]There are those who argue that because animals are sentient beings, they should not be harmed (Peter Singer, *Animal Liberation* [1975]). Some go further and claim that because they are sentient, animals have interests and therefore they have rights not to be harmed (Tom Reagan, *All That Dwell Therein* [1982]).

[28]Beckwith, *Politically Correct Death*, pp. 100-101.

[29]I am fully aware that very few would attempt such an argument today, but I am hopeful that it can be made someday.

[30]Thomson, "Defense," p. 131.

[31]Phillipa Foot, "The Problem of Abortion and the Doctrine of Double Effect"(1967), reprinted in *Moral Problems: A Collection of Philosophical Essays*, ed. by James Rachels (New York: Harper and Row, 1971), p. 29.

[32]Peter Kreeft, "Human Personhood Begins at Conception," Castello Institute Medical Ethics Policy Monograph (1995). Found at http://members.aol.com/pladvocate/person.html.

[33]Roland De Vaux, *Ancient Israel: Social Institutions*, Vol 1 (New York: McGraw Hill, 1965), p. 41.

[34]Scott Rae, *Moral Choices: An Introduction to Ethics* (Grand Rapids: Zondervan, 1995), p. 122.

[35]Rae, *Moral Choices*, pp. 122-123.

References

Books on Abortion

Bajema, Clifford E. *Abortion and the Meaning of Personhood.* Grand Rapids: Baker, 1974.

Beckwith, Francis J. *Politically Correct Death: Answering Arguments for Abortion Rights.* Grand Rapids: Baker, 1993.

_____, and Norman L. Geisler. *Matters of Life and Death: Calm Answers to Tough Questions about Abortion and Euthanasia.* Grand Rapids: Baker, 1991.

Lee, Patrick. *Abortion and Unborn Human Life.* Washington, DC: Catholic University of America Press, 1996.

Moreland, J.P. and Norman L. Geisler. *The Life and Death Debate.* Westport, CT: Praeger Books, 1990.

Pojman, Louis P. and Francis J. Beckwith. *The Abortion Controversy: A Reader.* Boston: Jones and Bartlett, 1994.

Schwartz, Stephen. *The Moral Question of Abortion.* Chicago: Loyola University Press, 1990.

Abortion Websites

The Abortion Law Home Page (http://members.aol.com/abtrbng/) A good source dealing with the current legal status of abortion on both the national and state level.

The Abortion Rights Activist Home Page (http://www.cais.com/agm/main/index.html) A pro-choice site with many articles, links, and an especially good reference section.

Ethics Updates: Abortion (http://ethics.acusd.edu/abortion.html) I consider "Ethics Updates" to be the best ethics website on the net. Put together by Lawrence Hinman, professor of philosophy at the University of San Diego, this site has almost everything on any topic in ethical theory or applied ethics. This is just one small part of his site that deals with abortion. Contains many sources from both sides of the argument.

FindLaw: Supreme Court Opinions (http://www.findlaw.com/casecode/supreme.html) Many bioethics issues determine or are concerned with important legal issues. This site provides an excellent search for any Supreme Court decision. You can get full text decisions or abstracts.

"Human Personhood Begins at Conception" (http://members.aol.com/pladvocate/person.html) A well-written article by Dr. Peter Kreeft, professor of philosophy at Boston College.

The Moral Question of Abortion by Stephen Schwartz (http://www.ohiolife.org/mqa/cover.htm) A rare find — a full book online. This is a well-written and tightly argued book for the pro-life position.

NOW and Abortion Rights/Reproductive Issues (http://www.now.org/issues/abortion/index.html) This is the National Organization of Women's page dealing with abortion and reproductive rights. Argues strongly for the pro-choice position.

The Ultimate Pro-Life List (http://www.prolife.org/ultimate/) Truly the ultimate site for pro-life discussions, resources, articles and other links. Very professional in appearance.

CHAPTER 3

A Good Death: Euthanasia

A Good Death: Euthanasia

Introduction
A. Definitions and Distinctions
  1. Definitions of Euthanasia and Death
    a. Failure of Heart and Lungs
    b. Separation of Body and Soul
    c. Whole Brain Death
    d. Neocortical Death
  2. Distinctions of Death and Euthanasia
    a. Active/Passive Distinction
    b. Withholding/Withdrawing Treatment
    c. Voluntary/Nonvoluntary Distinction
    d. The Ordinary/Extraordinary Means Distinction
B. The Legal Status of Euthanasia
  1. Karen Ann Quinlan
  2. Cruzan v. Missouri
C. Moral Arguments concerning Active Euthanasia
  1. Respect for Autonomy
  2. The Mercy Argument
  3. The Biographical/Biological Distinction
  4. The Bare Difference Argument
D. Passive Euthanasia
E. Other Issues Regarding End-of-Life Care
  1. Forgoing Nutrition and Hydration
  2. The Status of the PVS Patient
  3. Advanced Directives
F. Conclusion

3

By all accounts she was a free-spirited girl. Certainly her parents thought that. Her friends knew she played fast and loose claiming she was involved with drugs, though her parents denied it. On April 11, 1975, 21-year-old Karen Ann Quinlan moved out of her parents' house and rented a room with two male friends a few miles away. A few days later, April 14th, she joined one of her roommates, Thomas French, and a group of others to celebrate a friend's birthday at *Falconer's*, a local bar in the small North Jersey town of Lake Lacawanna. French reports that they had been drinking before the party and he had seen Karen "popping pills" earlier in the day. After a few drinks at the bar, the actual number is uncertain, Karen became dizzy and appeared faint. Her friends decided to take her home and let her sleep it off. By the time they had gotten her home she had completely passed out.

After putting her into bed, French decided to check on her about 15 minutes later. He discovered that she had stopped breathing. French performed mouth to mouth resuscitation while another roommate called the police. When the police arrived one took over the resuscitation efforts while the other questioned the two roommates. In their panic they lied and said that Karen was just staying over while her parents were on vacation and that they had simply found her having difficulty breathing. The police finally got her breathing again. Her color began to return, but she didn't regain consciousness.

Karen was transported to nearby Newton Memorial Hospital and admitted around midnight into the intensive care unit. In examining her possessions a bottle of Valium was discovered in her purse with some pills missing. Valium is a tranquilizer and, if mixed with alcohol or other drugs, it can be dangerous in slowing down the respiratory system causing anoxia, a loss of oxygen to the brain resulting in brain damage and often death. Karen had also been aggressively dieting, possibly even fasting, for several previous days. All of this may have contributed to Karen's condition, though the actual evidence of why she became initially unconscious is disputed.[1] Because of her difficulty breathing, Karen was placed on a small respirator for the first few days of her treatment. After nine days her condition had not changed and she was transferred to the larger St. Claires hospital in Denville, New Jersey which was staffed with neurologists that were not available at the smaller facility. Karen had difficulty with the smaller respirator and 4 days after admission was transferred to an MA-1 respirator which uses an intertracheal tube. A nasogastric tube was put in place for feeding purposes and she was placed on antibiotics.

Karen Ann Quinlan never regained consciousness. She was in a special coma-like state referred to today as persistent vegetative state. Her brain wave was not totally flat, but it was damaged to the point that it was believed she was not receiving any input from her senses. She would move her head, her eyes would remain open, she would even moan and make other vocal noises. But her body soon began to take on the rigidity found in most neurologically damaged patients and her weight dropped to 70-80 pounds.

Her family was understandably upset at her condition and were aware that her prognosis was hopeless. They were especially bothered in light of the fact that Karen had earlier shared with them her desire never to be kept alive in this condition. After three and a half months, and consulting with their family priest, they decided that this needed to end. Karen was dead for all intents and purposes. On July 31, 1975, they signed a release to have the respirator and nasogastric tubes removed.

Dr. Robert Morse initially agreed, but later backed down for a couple of reasons. First, St. Claires was a Catholic hospital and Morse was a Catholic himself. In those days many in the Catholic church thought that any form of euthanasia was equivalent to killing. Second, Morse consulted the hospital attorney who advised him not to disconnect Karen. Another important case had just concluded in Massachusetts in which a Dr. Eidolon was found guilty of criminal negligence for an unjustified late term abortion. The hospital lawyers thought the cases were too similar.

The Quinlans sought legal help from the local Legal Aid Society and found one in a young, idealistic lawyer, Paul Armstrong. Armstrong could have easily solved the case by simply asking the court to appoint Karen's father to be legal guardian. As legal guardian, Mr. Quinlan could have had Karen transferred to another hospital where they probably would have privately and discretely honored the family's wishes. However, Armstrong announced to the presiding judge, Robert Muir, that they were intending to remove Karen from the respirator and allow her to die. When Armstrong made that announcement, Judge Muir realized he could not appoint Mr. Quinlan as guardian. The legal guardian had to protect the interests of the patient. What Karen's interests were was now open to dispute because the issue of whether removal of treatment and allowing Karen to die was justified had not yet been established. Therefore Muir had no choice but to appoint a guardian *ad litem* (meaning "for the case"), a lawyer named Daniel Coburn, who would be an advocate for Karen. Armstrong was now forced to argue in court that Karen should be allowed to die. In making that announcement to the judge he set the stage for one of the most famous trials in the history of medical ethics: In the Matter of Karen Ann Quinlan.[2]

The word euthanasia is a combination of two Greek words: "*eu*" is the prefix for "good" and "*thanatos*" is the word for "death." Many today argue that for some people euthanasia can truly be a "good death" especially if they are suffering greatly or their lives are being unnecessarily prolonged by modern technology. Part of the confusion surrounding this issue is that the term "euthanasia" can be used a couple of different ways. In a narrow sense euthanasia can be defined as the intentional ending of a person's life, out of **motives** of either mercy, beneficence, or respect for personal autonomy. This has also been called "mercy killing." Under this definition, the aim of euthanasia is the death of the person to whom it is being applied. However, there is a broader definition of euthanasia which defines it as any act of relieving a person of the burdens of excessive medical treatment which one knows, with a high degree of reasonable probability, will result in the person's death. This definition is broader because it can incorporate the narrower view, but can also allow for actions where the death of the patient is not necessarily intended. In the early years of the euthanasia issue, the broader definition was employed. However in recent years the narrower definition seems to be the one most bioethicists mean. For our present purposes, whenever the term euthanasia is used without qualification, it will be referring to the broader definition.

Another term we need to discuss is **death**. A lot of controversy has been stirred up recently surrounding discussions of exactly when a person is considered to be dead. We first need to distinguish between definition of death and determination of death. Some will argue that it is the definition of death which needs to be reconsidered. However, the *definition* of death is not what is really being debated, but rather its *determination*. Death can be defined as the cessation of the essential characteristics and capacities that are necessary and sufficient conditions in order for a person to be alive. What are the "necessary and sufficient conditions" in order for a person to be alive? These can be discovered in examining the ways we have determined that someone is dead. Over time, four different concepts of determining death have been used.

Definitions and Distinctions

Four different concepts of determining death have been used.

1. *Failure of Heart and Lungs*. Throughout the majority of history the traditional determining factor for death has focused on the heart and lungs. When the breathing of air and the flow of blood have irreversibly stopped circulating, death has occurred. These are easily observed and even today most individuals are declared dead when circulation and respiration have ceased. Before the development of modern life-extending technologies, these were considered necessary and sufficient conditions for declaring death. With the advent of these machines, cessation of heart and lungs is no longer as decisive as it once was in determining death.

2. *Separation of Body and Soul*: Aristotle believed that the animating principle of life was the soul. Christianity takes a similar view and therefore defines death as when the soul leaves the body. For Christians the separation of soul and body is the necessary and sufficient condition for declaring someone dead. However, this is not observable and the question remains as to when specifically this occurs in the dying process. This is a theological truth and theological truths are difficult to defend empirically.

3. *Whole Brain Death*. **Whole brain death** is the absence and complete irrecoverability of all spontaneous brain activity and all spontaneous respiratory functions. This determination emerged when technological advances were able to intervene in the natural processes of heart and lung failure. Death is considered to have occurred when the entire brain has died. This is usually obtainable with the use of an electroencephalogram (EEG) which reads brain wave patterns. In 1968 an *ad hoc* committee at Harvard University established the first brain death standard. Called the *Harvard Criteria* it stated that if brain wave patterns are nearly or completely flat when administered twice over a 24 hour period, all brain activity

has ceased and the person is dead. In 1981 The President's Commission for the Study of Ethical Problems in Medicine and Biomedical and Behavioral Research established the Uniform Determination of Death Act. The act says:

> An individual who has sustained either (1) irreversible cessation of circulatory and respiratory functions, or (2) irreversible cessation of the entire brain, including the brain stem, is dead. A determination of death must be made in accordance with accepted medical standards.[3]

No one has ever survived brain death.

The UDDA is the standard determination of death today, and no one has ever survived brain death. However, some question whether this criterion for death is too narrow. They argue that this may be a sufficient criterion, but question if it is necessary. Is it possible that death could be determined before the whole brain is dead?

4. *Neocortical Death*. According to this criterion, a person is determined as dead when the outer layer of the brain covering the cerebrum, the neocortex, has irreversibly ceased to function. Because the functioning of the neocortex appears to be the biological precondition of consciousness, the result of its ceasing to function is the irreversible loss of consciousness and self-awareness, what some believe to be the primary basis for personhood. This is sometimes called "cerebral death," "higher brain death," or "apallic syndrome." Those patients who are deemed PVS (in a **persistent vegetative state**), such as Karen Ann Quinlan fit this description. There is much controversy over this determination of death. Though in 1986 the AMA recommended to accept **neocortical death** as an acceptable criterion for determining death, to date no state or federal government agency has accepted this standard. Thus neocortical death is viewed as a necessary condition for determining death, but at this time is not considered a sufficient condition.

Along with defining euthanasia and defining and determining death, we need to make some important distinctions. Again, it is because people have failed to make these distinctions that some confusion continues in the area of euthanasia.

1. *Active/Passive Distinction*. Of all the distinctions, this is the most important. Active euthanasia is the intentional and direct killing of another human life either out of motives of mercy, beneficence, or respect for personal autonomy. This is sometimes called mercy killing (our narrow definition above). This can be performed a number of ways: overdosing medication such as morphine, the use of violent means such as shooting or suffocating someone, or starving a patient to death. **Passive euthanasia** is the withholding or withdrawing of a life-sustaining treatment when certain justifiable conditions obtain and the patient is allowed to die from the debilitation or disease.

This is a very important distinction. There are two differences between these two types of acts. First is the difference of intention. In **active euthanasia** the intention or aim is to end the person's life. Should the person not die after the action is performed, the act would be deemed a failure. However, in passive euthanasia the intention is to relieve the patient of burdensome and unnecessary treatment. Should the patient not die, the act would not be deemed a failure because the patient would still be relieved of such treatment. Second, they are different in what is the direct cause of the patient's death. In active euthanasia the actions of the agent are what directly caused the patient's death: the agent killed him. In passive euthanasia it is not the action of the agent that is the direct cause of the patient's death, for example the removal of life-sustaining equipment, it is the debilitation or disease.

The distinction between active and passive euthanasia is not always clear to see.

This distinction is not always clear to see. One example might be to think of a healthy person on a respirator vs. a sick person on the respirator. If you take a normal healthy person and put them on a respirator, and then remove the respirator, nothing will happen to them because their normal respiratory system will continue to function spontaneously. However, if you take someone with a respiratory ailment and put him on a respirator and then remove him, he will die. What causes death in the second person is not the removal of the respirator. For if removing a person from a respirator causes death, then both persons would have died. It is the debilitation that causes death, and this is passive euthanasia. These days the debate is often framed in different terms. "Euthanasia" is used more for active euthanasia, while passive euthanasia is often referred to as "allowing one to die." As we shall see, there are those who want to erase this distinction altogether.

2. *Withholding/Withdrawing Treatment.* Withholding treatment simply means that treatment on a patient is never begun. Withdrawing Treatment is stopping treatment that has already begun. Some confuse this with active/passive euthanasia. Withholding seems passive and withdrawing seems active. This confusion was present in the New Jersey State Supreme Court case of Karen Ann Quinlan. However, they are not synonymous. There may be an emotional or psychological difference between these two actions. It may be psychologically more difficult to stop treatment than never to start it. However, there is really no morally relevant difference between them.

> *Withdrawing treatment is stopping treatment that has already begun.*

3. *Voluntary/Nonvoluntary/Involuntary Distinction.* Voluntary euthanasia occurs when a competent, informed patient autonomously requests it. This can be either while they are conscious or through an **advanced directive** like a **living will** or

durable power of attorney. Nonvoluntary euthanasia occurs whenever a person is incapable of forming a judgment concerning euthanasia and has left no advanced directive. The decision would have to be made for him by a third party based on what the third party would deem is in the best interest of the patient. Involuntary euthanasia occurs when a person expresses a desire to live but is killed or allowed to die. Of these three, the first and second **may** be justifiable under certain situations (see below). Involuntary euthanasia is never justified, even though there have been instances of it occurring. Herbert Hendlin reports of a case in the Netherlands (where euthanasia is tolerated) of a Catholic nun who specifically requested not to be euthanized as it was against her lifelong religious beliefs. The physician did so anyway claiming that she really wanted it, but "her religious convictions did not permit her to ask for death."[4] We will consider the Netherlands situation more fully in the next chapter.

4. *The Ordinary/Extraordinary Means Distinction*. This has been used as a way to classify treatment. **Ordinary means** has been used to describe all medicines, treatments, and procedures that offer a reasonable hope of benefit without placing undue burdens on a patient (pain or other serious inconvenience).

Extraordinary means has been used to describe those medicines, treatments, and procedures that are not ordinary because they involve excessive burdens on the patient and do not offer reasonable hope of benefit. In recent years these two terms have pretty much been abandoned. The problem was that they were just too vague and unspecific in a climate of constantly changing technology. "Reasonable hope" and "excessive burdens" change as technology changes. What was excessive years ago may be routine and ordinary today. Today bioethicists are more likely to think in terms of a benefits/burdens evaluation. Is the treatment providing enough of a benefit to offset the possible burdens? If the burdens outweigh the benefits, it is generally recommended that the treatment be withheld or withdrawn. It is important to note that such an evaluation cannot be made abstractly, but must be determined within specific contexts and with specific persons. While there are some medical standards based on the overall experience of the medical community, there are no universal or absolute guidelines for all treatments.

There have been two very important legal cases concerning euthanasia: Quinlan and Cruzan.

1. *In Re Karen Ann Quinlan* (1975, 1976). The case of Karen Ann Quinlan was the first euthanasia case to come before the courts. Some mark this event as the beginning of bioethics. There were actually two trials concerning Karen Ann Quinlan. The first trial took place in the Superior Court of New Jersey in Morristown. Judge Muir presided, Paul Armstrong argued for the Quinlans, and Daniel Coburn was advocate for Karen. Armstrong attempted first to argue that Karen was brain dead. Muir pointed out that the only standard for brain dead was whole brain death and this was not the case for Karen. Armstrong then tried to argue on the basis of "right to die." However, Muir pointed out that there was no precedent for such a right and the Constitution made no mention of it. Finally he settled on arguing right to privacy as determined in the *Griswold* case (see chapter 2). Coburn and the lawyers for the hospital argued that she was not brain dead, that there is always hope for some recovery, that there was no legal precedent for allowing Karen to die, and that removing her was equivalent to killing her. On Nov 10, 1975, almost seven months after Karen's lapsing into a comatose state, Judge Muir made his ruling. He ruled that (1) Karen was not brain dead; (2) Coburn was to remain the legal guardian of Karen; (3) any supposed prior directive or wishes expressed by Karen were unsubstantiated theoretical conversations and cannot be taken as final; (4) because Karen was incompetent and her wishes were not known, there was no violation of a right to privacy; (5) there is no constitutional "right to die"; and (6) a decision to terminate a respirator was a medical decision and therefore the doctors' decision.[5]

The Legal Status of Euthanasia

*Some mark the Quinlan case as
the beginning of bioethics.*

The Quinlan case was immediately appealed to the New Jersey State Supreme Court, bypassing all other appellate courts because of its precedent-setting implications. After several months of deliberation, The State Supreme Court ruled the following in January, 1976: (1) a patient's right to privacy was broad enough to encompass the right to decline medical treatment under certain circumstances; (2) right to privacy extends to an incompetent adult, and the guardian and family are permitted to assert the patient's right to privacy and render their best judgment; (3) ensuing death would not be ruled a homicide or suicide; (4) the lower court was right in not admitting prior statements by Karen as they were remote and lacked weight; (5) the lower court was also correct in denying removal of respirator, but was incorrect in denying guardianship to Mr. Quinlan; (6) life support may be terminated upon request of the family if physicians conclude there is "no reasonable probability" of return to a cognitive sapient state; (7) hospitals should form ethics committees to decide these types of issues in the future.

In handing down its decision, the State Supreme Court established the precedent for passive euthanasia that is in practice in every state in the country today. No longer are patients forced to remain chained to artificial machines in hopeless situations. However, it did not end so quickly for Karen. Even after the court's decision, and the Quinlan's official request to remove the respirator from Karen, the hospital refused to do so. By April she was still hooked up. Instead of disconnecting Karen from the respirator, which would have almost certainly meant her immediate death, they slowly "weaned" her off the respirator over a period of several weeks. Because of such weaning, Karen was finally able to breath spontaneously. In May 1976 she was moved out of the hospital and into a nursing home. She remained there until she finally died — *a full 10 years later* on June 13, 1986.

2. *Cruzan v. Director, Missouri Department of Health* (1990) On the night of January 11, 1983, 24-year-old Nancy Cruzan lost control of her car on a lonely stretch of Elm Road in Jasper County, Missouri. She was thrown 35 feet from the car and landed in a water-filled ditch. Paramedics found that her heart had stopped and she had not been breathing for at least 15 minutes. They were able to resuscitate her heart and lungs, but due to the anoxia, she was in a persistent vegetative state. Unlike Karen Ann Quinlan, Nancy could spontaneously breath so a respirator was not necessary. However, because she could not voluntarily swallow, she was connected up to a feeding tube inserted through her abdomen. After five years in this condition, Nancy's parents requested that the tube be removed and she be allowed to die. In the Quinlan case, the parents never requested that the feeding tube be removed so the issues of artificial feeding and nutrition had never been dealt with in court.

> *Before the Cruzan case, the issues of artificial feeding and nutrition had never been dealt with in court.*

The hospital was reluctant to remove the feeding tube, so the Cruzan's filed an appeal with the Jasper County Circuit Court who granted their request on July 27, 1988. However, the case was appealed to the Missouri State Supreme Court which reversed the lower court's decision. The court ruled that the state has a compelling interest in preserving life, regardless of quality of life, unless *clear and convincing evidence* of the patient's wishes concerning the end of life-sustaining treatment was available. Unfortunately Nancy had left no advanced directives, and parents' and friends' testimony recalling casual conversations in which Nancy said she would not want to be kept alive in "that" kind of state was deemed not clear and convincing evidence.

The Cruzan's appealed to the U.S. Supreme Court. This would be the first "right to die" case heard in the U.S. Supreme Court. The court heard the case on December 6, 1989, and announced their decision on June 25, 1990. They held the following: (1) The Missouri requirement for clear and convincing evidence was constitutional. States were allowed to determine their own standards of evidence. (2) A competent patient has the freedom to refuse medical treatment even if such refusal of treatment knowingly will cause death. This is not a "privacy" issue, but is a "liberty interest" issue. (3) In the case of incompetent patients, states are acting appropriately in requiring clear and convincing evidence of a patient's wishes, but such a standard is not federally mandated. (4) The withholding or withdrawing of artificial nutrition and hydration is no different then removal of other life-sustaining treatments.

Since the Supreme Court ruled that Missouri's standard of evidence was constitutional, the Cruzans were not able to remove the feeding tube from her. However, many of Nancy's friends did not testify in the original trial because they were unaware of the case at the time. Just before the accident occurred, Nancy had gotten a divorce. Most of her friends knew her as Nancy Davis, her married name. As they became aware of what had happened, they appealed to the court to reopen the case. When the state did so, it heard sufficient testimony to ascertain that Nancy indeed would have wanted to be allowed to die. On December 14, 1990, her feeding tube was removed, and Nancy died soon thereafter.

The Quinlan and Cruzan cases established the legal precedence for passive euthanasia and refusal of treatment.

The impact of both the Quinlan case and the Cruzan case was significant in regard to end-of-life care. They established the legal precedence for passive euthanasia and refusal of treatment in this country. It is now recognized that any person can refuse medical treatment at any time. As part of this right to refuse, it is also recognized that a person may request that burdensome treatment be removed and that they be allowed to die. However, these cases state nothing about active euthanasia and as of this writing, active euthanasia is recognized as murder in every state in the country.[6] The recent events surrounding Dr. Jack Kevorkian, undecided at the time of this writing, may have an impact on the issue of active euthanasia as distinct from the physician-assisted suicides for which he is better known.

While active euthanasia is, at this time, illegal, there are those who have argued for its legality. In general four moral arguments have been raised for the legitimacy of active euthanasia.

Moral Arguments concerning Active Euthanasia

1. *Respect for Autonomy*. Some have offered that persons should have the right to self-determination concerning all aspects of their lives, including the manner and time of their death. This idea is enveloped in the rhetoric of the right to die movement: "I have a right to choose to do what I want with my life. After all it is my life. If I choose to want to end it, that is my free choice. I am not hurting any other person." Margaret Battin argues for this point when she says that a physician respecting a patient's autonomy means, among other things, "providing the knowledge, equipment, and help to enable the patient to die if that is his or her choice; this is the other part of the physician's obligation, not yet recognized by the medical profession or the law of the United States."[7]

There are a number of problems here. First, this view of autonomy is too strong. It is simply too individual and independent. Philosopher Gilbert Meilaender calls this "excessive individualism." We are social creatures and one almost never acts in a manner that is completely and totally independent of others or which does not affect the community of which he or she is a part. Because we are social creatures, we have obligations to society. Even Cuban leader and atheist Fidel Castro recognized this. When one of the officials in his government committed suicide, he said, "Every revolutionary knows that he does not have the right to deprive his cause of a life that *does not belong to him,* and that he can only sacrifice against an enemy."[8] While it is true that as free creatures we do have the right of self-determination, it is a relative right not an absolute one. With our freedom comes responsibility to the community of which we are a part.

A second problem with the right-to-die argument is what many consider to be a coherency problem. Some question whether one can coherently have a natural right to die (the right to die being argued for must be a natural right, for a legal right to die has never been established). However, all natural rights presuppose our self-interested attachment to our own lives. In other words natural rights are rooted in the right to life, or in our natural self-preservation. For one to argue that one has a right to die is to argue that one has the right to annihilate the very basis of all rights including the right to die. Therefore, to propose such an annihilation would be ultimately self-defeating.[9]

Some question whether one can coherently have a natural right to die.

A third problem with the right-to-die argument has to do with the relationship between rights and obligations. All rights impose obligations on others. The fact that you have a right means others have some obligation to you concerning that right. Most rights are **negative rights** or rights of noninterference, which means that someone does not have the right to interfere with your choice. Those arguing for active euthanasia initially *seem* to be arguing for this kind of a right. However, they are actually asking for more than just to be left alone to die. They are not arguing for **suicide**; they are arguing for euthanasia, that is, for the right for others to kill them. This means they are arguing for a positive right which means that others, presumably physicians, will now have an obligation to kill patients. However, what of the physician's autonomy? What if he believes that killing others is wrong for religious or other reasons? If a patient has a *right* to euthanasia, then physicians now have an *obligation* placed on them to kill patients who request to die. Also since the physician now has an obligation to kill, it can be argued that he now also has a right to kill. Derail Charles points out the implications of this problem, "Should such a right be granted, what is to prevent the right to kill from being followed by the duty to kill? Will the 'right to die' only serve as the precursor to the duty to die?"[10]

If the argument from autonomy is valid, then one would have to argue that any autonomous individual has the right to die whether suffering or not.

Another problem with the autonomy argument is that, in the context of euthanasia, it is always coupled with suffering. If one is suffering enough, then one has the right to end one's life. However, if the argument from autonomy is valid and can really stand on its own, then one would have to argue that any autonomous individual at any time has the right to die and, as we argued, has the right to ask others to help. However, such a view is almost never argued for. Very few people would agree that a 22-year-old young woman, who has just gone through a divorce, recently lost her job, and believes that her life is meaningless, has the right to die. Even most suicide advocates would disagree that she has a right to die in this case. Yet if one agrees with the view of autonomy that is offered here, one must take this position to remain consistent.

Finally, as Christians we recognize that it is not *your* life. It is a gift from God, given to us only on loan, which we live in stewardship to Him. It simply is not ours to dispose of. Christian philosopher Gilbert Meilaender puts this best when he writes:

> What should be clear though, is that Christians do not approach this issue by first thinking in terms of a "right to life" or a "right to die with dignity." That is to say, we do not start with the language of independence. Within the story of my life I have the relative freedom of a creature, but it is not simply "my" life to do with as I please. I am free to end it, of course, but not free to do so without risking something as important to my nature as freedom: namely, the sense of myself as one who always exists in relation to God.[11]

2. *The Mercy Argument.* Returning to Margaret Battin, we find the principle of medical mercy to be, in part, "Where possible one ought to relieve the pain and suffering of another person, when it does not contravene that person's wishes . . . [and] where it will not violate other moral obligations. . . ."[12] Battin holds, as do others, that at times this principle will require euthanasia. The most common illustration used to support this principle is our treatment of injured animals. Out of compassion, we often kill animals to put them out of their misery, surely we should show the same compassion to persons as well. Doctors have an obligation to end suffering and mercifully bringing about death can be one way to fulfill this obligation.

A number of responses could be made to this argument. First, we need to separate pain and suffering. By pain I am referring primarily to a physical condition in a person while suffering generally entails a broader concept involving a number of psychological factors as well as physical pain. As far as pain is concerned, much has been done in the area of pain management. In the past two decades we have seen tremendous advancements in medications and palliative treatment for pain. Dr. Matthew E. Connolly reports that:

> In the truly good centers of palliative care, such as St. Christopher's Hospice in London, they control cancer pain in

95% of the patients they see. In the 5% where less than ideal control is accomplished, it is usually because the patients were presented too late for everything to be done before death occurs.[13]

He argues that much still needs to be done. The number one problem in pain management is education. One of the fears Dr. Connolly has is that, with the present acceptance of active euthanasia and physician-assisted suicide, there will be less of an emphasis on the need for education and research in pain management. In the next chapter we will see this fear is justified in examining what is occurring in the Netherlands.

Suffering involves more than just physical pain. It involves psychological states that may or may not also involve physical pain. Many people fear loss of control, depression, anxiety, and loneliness more than they fear the physical suffering itself. Rather than confirming their worst fears by encouraging active euthanasia, we need to be meeting these needs through caring relationships. Dr. Martha Twaddle comments that "A good patient-physician relationship is worth 10mg of morphine, as presence alone can ease the anguish of fear."[14] She recommends Hospice care, a relatively new form of holistic medicine dealing specifically with those who are dying. Hospice rejects the active euthanasia model and adopts a model of dealing with the total pain and suffering of the patient. The goal is to accompany patients in the dying process, easing the journey with medications, explanation and presence.

A second response to the mercy argument is that it communicates the wrong message about pain and suffering. Suffering is a natural part of the human experience. It is part of life, a means of growth, and it shouldn't necessarily be avoided at *all costs*. I am not advocating that we should actively seek suffering or even rejoice in its presence. We should do all we can to relieve suffering, but we shouldn't think we can do absolutely anything to relieve suffering. Just because one is suffering, it doesn't mean any action is now justified for the cause of the relief of suffering. Dr. Marsha Fowler writes that the answer in dealing with the suffering patient is not in mastering suffering with medicine, avoiding

it through euthanasia, or even explaining it theologically;
"Rather the answer is in facing the experience of suffering."[15]
This is specifically why the analogy with an animal breaks
down. It isn't just that humans have a value that animals do
not share (which I believe is true and is why killing an animal
is not the same as killing a person). But more importantly,
humans are persons with the ability to rationally reflect upon
the nature of their circumstances, to reflect on who they are,
and what kind of person they want to be. They can respond
to suffering in a positive way that an animal cannot. H.
Richard Niebuhr said it best: "It is in response to suffering
that many and perhaps all [persons]. . . define themselves,
take on character, develop their ethos."[16]

---

*The mercy argument communicates the
wrong message about pain and suffering.*

For Christians suffering has an even deeper meaning. Gilbert
Meilaender states this deeper meaning well:

> We remember, after all, that Jesus goes to the cross in the
> name of obedience to his Father. We need not glorify or seek
> suffering, but we must be struck by the fact that a human
> being who is a willing sufferer stands squarely in the center of
> Christian piety. Jesus bears his suffering not because it is
> desirable but because the Father allots it within the limits of
> his earthly life.[17]

While we need to care for those who are suffering, and not
kill them, we must remember that we cannot always relieve it
and even God won't always take it away. But God under-
stands suffering; he has lived through it himself in the person
of Jesus Christ. "God himself lives that problem and bears it.
His way is steadfast love through suffering, and it is the mystery of God's own being and power that this truly proves to
be the way to maximize care for all who suffer."[18]

3. *The Biographical/Biological Distinction.* This argument and the one below come from philosopher James Rachels. They both have been very influential in the euthanasia debate. This particular argument draws a distinction between a human organ's biological life and a person's biographical life. A biologically living being has no moral status. All living beings fit into this category: animals, plants, etc. Moral status is granted only to a human being with a biographical life. What makes up a biographical life? Rachels claims it is, "the sum of one's aspirations, decisions, activities, projects, and human relationships"[19] Some types of humans do not have biographical lives. Infants have not had one yet. Certain comatose humans no longer have one. These people do not have any real moral status at all. He also places certain persons in this category who are competent and functioning as human person's. He uses the famous case of Dax Cowart, a young man who was severely burned in a gas explosion and who continually requested to be allowed to die but was kept under treatment in a hospital for about two years against his will. Rachels argues that because Dax can no longer live the active kind of life he used to live, that he has lost his "biographical life" and should be euthanized.

> *Human beings have intrinsic value simply because they are human beings.*

We might have a number of responses to Rachels's distinction between the biological and biographical.[20] First, any concept of biographical life has to presuppose the importance of a biological human life. A "biographical life" is what we have called in other parts of this book personhood. We have already seen that biological human organisms are by nature of what they are, persons. It is a thing's nature that determines what kind of thing it is (dog, tree, human person). It is the fact that you have a human nature that makes you a human being. Conversely, a biographical life is only possible because it is grounded in a human being that can biologically have that kind of life. Therefore the biological life is morally just as important as the biographical life. Human beings have intrinsic value simply because they are human beings.

Second, even if we grant Rachels's distinction, he assumes that a biologically living thing has no moral status, only persons. However, a thing doesn't have to be a person to have moral status in the sense of how it is treated. There are many nonpersonal things we say have intrinsic value and therefore cannot be treated any way one wishes. For example, artwork has this kind of value. Many would argue that the Mona Lisa or Michelangelo's statue of David have value of themselves. It would be immoral for a person to destroy or disfigure them, not just because of their monetary or social value, but because they have intrinsic value being the created works of human beings. Also, we place a certain value on other sentient beings saying it would be immoral to torture or treat them cruelly. A third example would be future generations. Many argue that we have an obligation to future generations to guarantee that they have a safe and pleasant environment to live in. Yet these persons do not even exist. Therefore, it goes against our experience to argue that only persons have moral status. Human organisms may be in the same category of these things, and therefore you can't just treat them any way you wish.

Third, Rachels's conception of the biographical life is too broad and subjective. Rachels defines it merely as a person's "aspirations, decisions, activities, projects, and human relationships." This means a person is free to choose whatever goals, interests and desires that are important to him with no standards at all. They then may claim that when the capacity to participate in these interests is no longer available, their biographical life is gone and they should be allowed to die. An example of this kind of thinking is in the play, and later film, *Whose Life Is It Anyway?* The story is told of a sculptor who is involved in an auto accident and paralyzed from the neck down. He will no longer be able to do sculpting, which was his life. The playwright takes Rachels's position in saying that the sculptor should be allowed to die. However, just because a person is restricted from doing what they are interested in, does that mean it would be morally justifiable for them to be killed upon request? Isn't it possible that the sculptor could still have a meaningful life? The lives of victims of tragic accidents such as Christopher Reeve and Joni Erickson Tada show that a meaningful life is possible even after the tragedy.

Fourth, if this distinction is valid, then a person who has lost his biographical life is no longer a person and therefore loses all other moral rights as well. This means it might be possible to perform medical experiments on him or kill him in a violent and brutal fashion. Since we are no longer dealing with an object with moral rights, in the absence of other ethical factors, you are free to treat such a person any way you wish.

4. *The Bare Difference Argument.* This argument, also from Rachels, is an attempt to erase the distinction between active and passive euthanasia by showing they both result in the same end. It states that the active/passive distinction is a distinction without a difference. There is no difference between intentionally killing someone and allowing someone to die — in the end they are both dead as the result of your actions or your failure to act. Therefore, the conclusion is that if passive euthanasia is sometimes justifiable, then active euthanasia is sometimes justifiable. Rachels has produced a well-known story to illustrate this argument. It is called "The Boy in the Bathtub" illustration and I have summarized it here:

> Two men, Smith and Jones, both stand to inherit millions upon the deaths of their six-year-old cousins. Smith plans to kill his cousin and sneaks into the bathroom while he is bathing. He holds his head under water until he drowns. Jones also plans to kill his cousin. He sneaks into the bathroom intending to drown him. However, before he gets to him, the boy slips and hits his head, and he sinks into unconsciousness before going under water. Jones does nothing but just stands there and watches the boy drown ready to push him back under if necessary, but the boy never comes back up. Thus Smith killed his cousin, but Jones merely allowed his cousin to die. However, we would hold that both of these men are morally despicable. Therefore, there is no real difference between killing and allowing someone to die.[21]

A number of philosophers have had problems with Rachels's illustration. Dr. James Childress comments that, "Rachels's examples may not be as conclusive as he thinks. Smith's and Jones's vicious motives may obscure other features of the case which might be important in other settings . . . his case throws no light on our dilemmas in the use of biomedical technology. These dilemmas arise precisely because we do not know what constitutes 'doing good' for patients in all cases."[22] Childress's point is that Rachels's illustration is about persons doing bad, but it doesn't necessarily apply to people trying to do good.

Dr. J.P. Moreland points out that the real problem with Rachels's illustration is that it presents an inadequate analysis of moral actions.[23] Moral acts are more than just the movement of body parts. Moral acts have to take into account motive and intention as well as the means to an action. Of the three, intention is where the real essence of the moral act lies. "The Boy in the Bathtub" illustration differs only in means to an end (killing vs. allowing to die), but the motive and intention are the same (both Smith and Jones desire and intend to have their cousin die). While Smith may be legally charged with murder while Jones is not, we hold them both morally responsible. In active euthanasia the intention is the death of the patient. In passive euthanasia the intention is the relief of the patient from excessive burdens with the knowledge that this will most probably, though not necessarily, result in the patient's death.

> *Moral acts are more than just the movement of body parts.*

None of the arguments in favor of active euthanasia are as strong as they first appear, and certainly none of them justify killing another person. We will finish this section with the following quote by Gilbert Meilaender about Paul Ramsey, one of the truly great Christian ethicists:

In a chapter written a quarter century ago that remains to this day a classic discussion of the issues, Paul Ramsey sought to articulate an ethic of "(only) caring for the dying." Such an ethic he suggested, would reject two opposite extremes: refusing to acknowledge death by continuing the struggle against it when that struggle is useless, or aiming to hasten the coming of death. Neither of these can count as *care* for one of our fellow human beings; each is a form of abandonment. We should always try to care for the dying person, but we should only care. To try to do more by seizing either extremes is always to give something other or less than care.[24]

Passive Euthanasia

We have argued that active euthanasia is not justified because it is actively and intentionally taking another life. We have also argued that there is a distinction between active and passive euthanasia. The question to address now is: Is passive euthanasia ever justifiable? The answer to that is a qualified yes. It may be justifiable in certain situations when certain conditions hold. What would the conditions be? Most ethicists recognize the following: (1) the patient is terminal, meaning that he/she is in the latter stages of the dying process; (2) death is imminent and/or treatment is futile; (3) treatment is excessively burdensome with little benefit; (4) death is not directly intended and the action taken is not the direct cause of death; (5) the patient has autonomously requested or agreed to the action. Two comments about these conditions are in order. First, they do not all have to hold, though most of them should be present. The "intention" aspect of the fourth condition is the most important aspect and must be present. The intention in passive euthanasia is always to relieve the patient of excessively burdensome treatment, not to cause the patient's death, even though this may be a foreseen consequence. Second, there is some debate about some of these conditions. Some believe that the fifth condition is not absolute if the patient has not left any directives. One can use a "best interest" standard in deciding to allow a patient to die if the other conditions are in place. In addition, some hold that death must be imminent under the second condition while others recognize that futility plays a role in this decision as well. Death was not imminent for Karen Ann Quinlan, but her condition was futile.

One of the more controversial discussions concerns the fourth condition. Some believe that, as long as the intention is right, the action taken may be the direct cause of death. In other words if you give a lethal dose of morphine to a patient with the intention of relieving suffering knowing that it will kill the patient, it is not considered active euthanasia because your intention was not to kill, but to relieve suffering. Those who hold this position often say it is an application of the **principle of double effect**.[25] Others say that this is an incorrect application of the principle, because the first condition of the principle says that the action one is doing must be "either good or at least morally neutral." However, giving a patient a lethal dose of medication is neither good nor morally neutral, it is evil itself. Therefore double effect doesn't apply to this action.

The major argument in favor of passive euthanasia is that it is a recognition that medical science can only do so much.

The major argument in favor of passive euthanasia is that it is a recognition that medical science can only do so much, and that one must recognize this and allow death to come at the proper time. This is not killing someone, it is a recognition that there is nothing more we can do to keep the person alive. As Paul Ramsey said, a time comes when we need to stop "struggling against death" by any means possible. Along with this argument, we can argue that because death is not intended and the action is not causing death, a mistaken diagnosis would not be failure. The person could get well, or at least survive, and this would not be deemed a tragedy. No such possibility exists with active euthanasia.

Before leaving the topic of euthanasia, there are three other issues to be addressed.

1. *Forgoing Nutrition and Hydration.* As we saw in the Cruzan case, the Supreme Court deemed that removal of artificial nutrition and hydration should be treated like any other medical treatment. However, while that settles the legal question, there is still an ethical question to be addressed: Should the administering of artificially induced food and water be handled in the same way as other medical treatments in the consideration of passive euthanasia? In other words, can they be withdrawn from a terminally ill patient in much the same way as other medical intervention might be withdrawn?

> *In passive euthanasia, it is the disease which is the direct cause of death.*

There is some division among Christian philosophers on this issue. Dr. J.P. Moreland, Dr. Norman Geisler, and Dr. Gilbert Meilaender have all argued that, in most cases, nutrition and hydration should not be treated as the same as other treatments and therefore should not be removed.[26] They cite the following as reasons: (1) Medical treatment is performed for therapeutic reasons to treat some disease. Food and water do not have as their purpose the treatment of disease; they are for the sustaining of life. (2) In passive euthanasia, it is the disease which is the direct cause of death, not the action taken by the health care worker. If artificial hydration and nutrition are withdrawn, that direct action is what will result in the patient's death. This is active euthanasia. (3) In withdrawing or withholding extraordinary life-sustaining treatment (passive euthanasia), the focus is on the quality of the treatment. The purpose is to spare a person an unduly burdensome means of medical intervention. However, in withdrawing or withholding food and water (active euthanasia), the focus shifts from the quality of the treatment to the quality of the patient's life itself. (4) There are three criteria in which withholding or withdrawing nutrition and hydration might be justified: If the person is going to die in a very short time whether or not he has nutrition and hydration; death is not intended nor directly caused by the forgoing of nutrition or hydration; the means of administering food and water was excessively burdensome and extraordinary.

Other Christian philosophers believe that in some cases, most often the PVS case, artificial nutrition and hydration may be justifiably removed. Dr. Scott Rae seems more open to this view. He writes, "If one admits that this is indeed genuine medical treatment, and if one allows some place for **substituted judgment**, then removal of nutrition and hydration can be ethically justified apart from any considerations of personhood."[27] However, he says that certain conditions must be met before removing artificial nutrition and hydration: (1) it is medically determined that the patient cannot absorb nutrients; (2) the burdens outweigh the benefits; (3) there is no reasonable hope for the patient to regain consciousness; (4) the patient has left an advanced directive concerning her desires should she end up in this situation. Another Christian who argues for removal of food and water is Dr. Robert Rakestraw. We will look at his argument below.

2. *The Status of the PVS Patient.* Another area where there is disagreement even among Christians is the status of the PVS patient. In order to understand this disagreement, one needs to understand what persistent vegetative state means. A persistent vegetative state (PVS) is a condition of permanent unconsciousness in which the person is completely unaware of himself or his surroundings though he may appear to be awake and go through regular sleep/wake cycles. It is usually the result of permanent neocortical impairment and is considered irreversible. PVS patients may exhibit many lower-brain stem functions: they usually do not need life-sustaining treatment with the exception of a feeding tube, breathe spontaneously, have a regular heartbeat, digest normally, experience grasp reflex, chew, yawn and even groan and make other vocal

sounds. However, it is fairly well established that all capacity for consciousness, self-awareness, memory, personality, communication and sentience are irreversibly lost. People in this state can exist as long as 30 years in this condition. PVS is not the same as a coma, which is a sleep-like state that is potentially reversible, "locked-in" syndrome where the patient is conscious but is unable to communicate orally, or whole brain death.

> *Rakestraw holds that personhood is present from the moment of conception until these abilities or potentials cease.*

Many persons believe that because the neocortex is the seat of the capacities for the functioning of personhood, and because the neocortex is irreversibly dead, that therefore the person is dead and all that is left alive is the human organism. Christian theologian Dr. Robert Rakestraw adopts this view. Rakestraw holds the view of personhood similar to the one we defended in the last chapter. As a person man is made in the image of God "with the actual ability or potential to be aware of oneself and to relate in some way to one's environment, to other human beings, and to God."[28] He holds that personhood is present from the moment of conception until these abilities or potentials cease. In the language we used in the last chapter, personhood ceases when the basic inherent capacity of personhood ceases to be present. He writes:

> It appears, then, that neocortical destruction equals the end of personal life because the correctly diagnosed PVS individual is a body of organs and systems, artificially sustained without the personal human spirit that once enabled this body-soul unity to represent God on earth. Since the Bible on occasion uses the language of the human spirit's departure — as something different from a person's life-force or final breath — to signify death (Luke 23:46; Acts 7:59-60), we may use similar language in suggesting that the spirit of the PVS individual has already returned to God.[29]

It is important to understand Rakestraw's argument here. He is *not* claiming that the immediate capacities for personhood are merely not functioning, he is claiming that the basic inherent capacity is no longer present. Therefore the person is gone. Rakestraw also believes that recent breakthroughs have been made which have made the determination of neocortical irreversibility virtually certain. Medical scientists now have a test, called a positron emissions tomographic (PET) test, to distinguish between coma, "locked-in" syndrome and complete neocortical death making misdiagnosis more improbable. Some argue that if we do not recognize neocortical death as the death of the person, then we will be forced to keep thousands of bodies alive for several years with no hope of functioning as persons. The longest case of PVS is 37 years. Rakestraw would argue that we can remove artificial hydration and nutrition from PVS patients and allow them to die, since they are not persons.

The longest case of PVS is 37 years.

A number of Christian philosophers disagree with Rakestraw's conclusion concerning the status of the PVS patient. Dr. J.P. Moreland states that, "If there is evidence that a holistic living organism is present, then the human soul is present."[30] He takes the PVS patient to be a full person. Dr. Scott Rae also disagrees with Rakestraw and others who hold to neocortical death as the death of the person. Dr. Rae refers to Rakestraw's position as a "functional view" as opposed to an "essential" view of personhood, and considers such a view as "dangerous."[31] While I agree that a functional view of personhood is dangerous, I believe that Dr. Rae has misunderstood the thrust of Rakestraw's position. He is not saying that the PVS patient is simply not *functioning* as a person, but that he has lost the *basic inherent capacity* to function as one. In other words, Rakestraw is claiming that, what Dr. Moreland described in our last chapter as "a fairly standard set of highest order of capacities for mental states" that "constitute" personhood is no longer present. Whether one agrees with Rakestraw or not, it would be wrong to place him in the same functionalistic camp as Feinberg and Warren.

Those who believe that PVS patients should not be disconnected from artificial nutrition and hydration usually cite three reasons: (1) These persons are not biologically dead. The heart and lungs are functioning normally and brain death has not occurred. They are still living human beings. (2) There are cases, though rare, of patients diagnosed as PVS who have spontaneously recovered, some having been in this state as long as six months. (3) Food and water are not extraordinary care, but are ordinary care for these patients. At this point two things have been legally acknowledged: No state has accepted neocortical death as a legal standard for death, and artificial nutrition and hydration is a form of medical treatment and can, with the patient's or surrogate's permission, be removed just like any other treatment.

3. *Advanced Directives*. An advanced directive is a set of instructions from a competent, autonomous, informed person regarding decisions about future medical treatment in the event that the person becomes incapable of making a decision at a future time. An advanced directive expresses the person's desires regarding medical treatments and can designate a surrogate decision-maker. Many states require all hospitals to inform patients concerning their rights to refuse treatment and concerning advanced directives upon admission. Advanced directives are an important safeguard in our age of modern life-saving technology.

An advanced directive is instruction regarding decisions about future medical treatment.

There are two basic types of advanced directives. First, there are living wills. A living will is simply a document that expresses an individual's preferences for treatment. In many states you do not even need an attorney to create a living will as long as there are at least two persons who can witness the will. It is important to note that even after signing a will, a person still has the right to make health care decisions as long as he is able. You are not locked into the will if you are still competent to state your desires. Also, living wills are often intentionally vague so that they can meet all kinds of situations.

The second form of advanced directive is the durable power of attorney. This is a person, designated in advance by the patient, to act as a proxy decision-maker at the time that the patient is no longer able to make decisions concerning his own welfare. This is more flexible than a living will and therefore is generally preferable. A person can be more sensitive to changing circumstances and can clarify the wishes of the patient. Despite the title, they do not have to be an attorney. They are usually a close family member.

While either of these forms of advanced directives are preferable to nothing, the best form of advanced directive is a combination of both. The living will can give your stated preferences and the person in the role of durable power of attorney can help interpret these to the specific situation and make sure they are carried out. I would advise all to have some form of advanced directive.

Conclusion   The Christian philosopher Gilbert Meilaender wrote, in a well-known essay on euthanasia, "Life is a great good, but not the greatest good (which is fidelity to God)."[32] In that sentence he sums up the twofold response that we as Christians must have toward euthanasia.

One response is the recognition that life has an end called death. Death is not something we eagerly seek, but it is not something to be avoided at all costs. God has appointed the limits of our life and we must accept them. Meilaender writes, "Recognizing our life as a trust we will be moved not by an 'absolute will to live' but a will to live within these limits."[33] Part of the recognition of such limits is to allow persons to die when that time has come and not require that they be endlessly attached to tubes and machines.

The other response is, in recognizing that fidelity to God is the highest good, we need to be faithful to him in allowing him to impose the limits on this life, and not take it upon ourselves to do it. It is not our role to bring on death; that role belongs to God alone. "We are tempted to be 'like God' when we toy with the possibility of defining our love — and the meaning of humanity — apart from the appointed limits of human life."[34] One of the limits that God has placed upon us is that we are not to kill other human beings. Meilaender continues:

> This vision of the world and of the meaning of life and death, has within Christendom given guidance to those reflecting on human suffering and dying. That moral guidance has amounted to the twofold proposition that, though we might properly cease to oppose death . . . we ought never aim at death as either our end or our means.[35]

Both of our responses, to allow life to end but never to hasten its ending, flow out of Christian love. Some may argue that active euthanasia is done from love. While one who euthanizes may indeed do so out of compassion, I would offer that Christian love would not lead one to hasten another's death. "Such action cannot be loving because it cannot be part of the meaning of commitment to the well-being of another human being within the appointed limits of earthly life. . . . it is not the creaturely love which Christians praise, a love which can sometimes do no more than suffer as best we can with the sufferer."[36]

There is a distinction between minimizing suffering and maximizing love.

In short, there is a distinction between minimizing suffering and maximizing love. Those who advocate active euthanasia often confuse this distinction. We should try to minimize suffering within the limits we can, but we should never go outside of those limits. A final comment by Meilaender is appropriate to close this discussion:

> In that Christian world, in which death and suffering are great evils but not the greatest evil, love can never include in its meaning hastening a fellow human being toward [the evil of] death, nor can it mean a refusal to acknowledge death when it comes [as an evil but not the greatest evil]. We can only know what the imperative "maximize love" means if we understand it against the background assumptions which make intelligible for Christians words like 'love' and 'care.' The Christian mind has certainly not recommended that we seek suffering or call it an unqualified good, but it is an evil which when endured faithfully, can be redemptive.[37]

ENDNOTES

[1]Contradictory evidence exists of what the initial toxicology screen reported about Karen. The attending physician said there was a small amount of barbiturates in her system; a consulting neurologist said there was evidence of quinine, Valium, and Librium, but no evidence for morphine or barbiturates, and her parents claim that the early reports showed only normal "therapeutic" levels of aspirin and Valium in her system. From Gregory Pence, *Classic Cases in Medical Ethics* (New York: McGraw Hill, 1990).

[2]Details concerning Karen Ann Quinlan's story were gathered through various sources including Pence, *Classic Cases*, pp. 9-11 and Merrill Sheils, "Who was Karen Quinlan?" *Newsweek* (86 Nov 3, 1975), p. 60.

[3]The President's Commission for the Study of Ethical Problems in Medicine and Biomedical and Behavioral Research, *Defining Death: Medical, Legal, and Ethical Issues in the Definition of Death* (Washington, DC: U.S. Government Printing Office, 1981), p. 159.

[4]Herbert Hendlin, *Seduced by Death: Doctors, Patients and Assisted Suicide* (New York: W.W. Norton, 1998), p. 20.

[5]In Re Karen Quinlan, 348 A.2d 801; Superior Court of New Jersey.

[6]Recognized legal and moral distinctions exist between euthanasia and physician-assisted suicide. We will discuss these distinctions in the next chapter. The latter has been legalized in the state of Oregon.

[7]Margaret Pabst Battin, *The Least Worst Death: Essays in Bioethics on the End of Life* (New York: Oxford University Press, 1994), p. 113.

[8]Cited in Michael Walzer, *Obligations* (New York: Simon & Schuster, 1970), p. 172.

[9]This argument can be found in Leonard Kass, "Is There a Right to Die?" *Hastings Center Report* (Jan-Feb, 1993), p. 36.

[10]Derail Charles, "The Right to Die in the Light of Contemporary Rights Rhetoric," in *Bioethics and the Future of Medicine: A Christian Appraisal*, ed. by John F. Kilner, Nigel de S. Cameron, and David L. Scheidermeyer (Grand Rapids: Eerdmans, 1995), p. 272.

[11]Gilbert Meilaender, *Bioethics: A Primer for Christians* (Grand Rapids: Eerdmans, 1996), p. 60.

[12]Battin, *Least Worst Death*, p. 101.

[13]Matthew E. Connolly, "The Management of Cancer Pain," in *Suicide: A Christian Response* (Grand Rapids: Kregel Publications, 1998), p. 94.

[14]Martha L. Twaddle, "Hospice Care," in *Death with Dignity: A Christian Appraisal* (Grand Rapids: Eerdmans, 1996), p. 186.

[15]Marsha D.M. Fowler, "Suffering," in *Death with Dignity*, p. 50.

[16]Richard H. Niebuhr, *The Responsible Self* (New York: Harper and Row, 1963), p.60.

[17]Gilbert Meilaender, "Euthanasia and Christian Vision"(1982), reprinted in *On Moral Medicine: Theological Perspectives in Medical Ethics*, ed. by Stephen Lammers and Allen Verhey (Grand Rapids: Eerdmans, 1987), p. 457.

[18]Meilaender, *Bioethics*, p. 66.

[19]James Rachels, *The End of Life* (New York: Oxford University Press, 1986), p. 5.

[20]I am indebted to my friend and colleague Dr. J.P. Moreland for his analysis and critique of Rachels's arguments. I am borrowing much of my material from his book, *The Life and Death Debate: Moral Issues of our Time*, with Norman L. Geisler (Westport CT: Greenwood Press, 1990).

[21]James Rachels, "Active and Passive Euthanasia" (1975) reprinted in Gregory Pence, *Classic Works in Medical Ethics* (New York: McGraw Hill, 1998), p. 24.

[22]James F. Childress, *Priorities in Biomedical Ethics* (Philadelphia: Westminster, 1981), p. 37.

[23]Moreland, *Life and Death Debate*, pp. 75-76.

[24]Meilaender, *Bioethics*, p. 62. The work by Ramsey that he is referring to is chapter 3 of Ramsey's classic, *The Patient as Person* (New Haven, CT: Yale University Press, 1970).

[25]The principle of double effect has a long and controversial history within Christian Ethics. It originates within the writings of Thomas Aquinas and basically says that one action can have two effects — one good and one evil. As long as the good effect was the intended effect, the evil effect does not account against one. There are actually four conditions to the principle of double effect: (1) the intended act itself must be morally good or at least morally neutral; (2) the agent may not intend the bad effect, but he may foresee it and allow it to take place; (3) the good effect must be produced directly by the agent's intended action and not by the unintended bad effect; (4) the intended effect must be proportionately good to compensate for allowing the unintended, though perhaps foreseen, bad effect. My point in the body of the chapter is that while conditions 2-4 are met, some believe, myself included, that the first condition is violated when one knowingly gives a patient a lethal dose of medication. One may

argue that we are simply giving medicine and avoid the terminology of "lethal dose." This would be possible if we really do not know if the dosage we are giving is actually lethal or not, it just may be. If that is the case then the principle of double effect may apply. But if one has good reason to believe that the dosage will be lethal, I don't believe he can appeal to the principle of double effect.

[26]See Moreland, *Life and Death Debate*, pp. 78-80; for Dr. Geisler see *Matters of Life and Death* (Grand Rapids: Baker, 1999), pp. 142-143; for Dr. Meilaender see his "On Removing Food and Water: Against the Stream," *Hastings Center Report* 14 (December 1984), pp. 11-13.

[27]Scott Rae, *Moral Choices: An Introduction to Ethics* (Grand Rapids: Zondervan, 1995), p. 177.

[28]Robert. V. Rakestraw, "The Persistent Vegetative State and the Withdrawal of Nutrition and Hydration" (1992), reprinted in *Readings in Christian Ethics*, ed. by David K. Clark and Robert V. Rakestraw (Grand Rapids: Baker, 1996), p.127.

[29]Rakestraw, "Persistent Vegetative State," p. 128.

[30]J.P. Moreland, personal correspondence, December 16, 1998.

[31]Rae, *Moral Choices*, p. 176.

[32]Gilbert Meilaender, "Euthanasia and Christian Vision," p. 457

[33]Ibid., pp. 456-457.

[34]Ibid., p. 459.

[35]Ibid., p. 457.

[36]Ibid.

[37]Ibid., p. 458.

References

Sources Dealing with Euthanasia

Battin, Margaret Pabst. *The Least Worst Death: Essays in Bioethics on the End of Life*. New York: Oxford University Press, 1994.

Beckwith, Francis J. and Norman L. Geisler. *Matters of Life and Death*. Grand Rapids: Baker, 1999.

Beauchamp, Tom L., ed. *Intending Death: The Ethics of Assisted Suicide and Euthanasia*. Upper Saddle River, NJ: Prentice-Hall, 1996.

Beauchamp, Tom L. and Robert M. Veatch. *Ethical Issues in Death and Dying*. 2nd ed. Upper Saddle River, NJ: Prentice-Hall, 1996.

Kilner, John F., Arlene B. Miller, and Edmund D. Pellegrino. *Dignity and Dying: A Christian Appraisal*. Grand Rapids: Eerdmans, 1996.

Larson, E.J and D.W. Admunsen. *A Different Death: Euthanasia and the Christian Tradition*. Downers Grove, IL: InterVarsity, 1998.

Moreland, J.P. and Norman L. Geisler. *The Life and Death Debate: Moral Issues of Our Time*. Westport, CT: Greenwood Press, 1990.

Moreno, Jonathan D. *Arguing Euthanasia*. New York: Touchstone (Simon and Schuster), 1995.

Rakestraw, Robert V. "The Persistent Vegetative State and the Withdrawal of Nutrition and Hydration" (1992). Reprinted in *Readings in Christian Ethics*. Ed. by David K. Clark and Robert V. Rakestraw. Grand Rapids: Baker, 1996.

Stewart, Gary P. et al. *Basic Questions on Suicide and Euthanasia: Are They Ever Right?* Grand Rapids: Kregel, 1998.

Uhlmann, Michael M., ed. *Last Rights: Assisted Suicide and Euthanasia Debated*. Grand Rapids: Eerdmans, 1998.

Wekessor, Carol. *Euthanasia: Opposing Viewpoints*. Westport, CT: Greenwood Press, 1995.

Websites Dealing with Euthanasia

Citizens United for Resisting Euthanasia (http://pw2.netcom.com/~cureltd/index.html) An anti-euthanasia organization with many anti-euthanasia and anti-suicide articles.

Compassion in Dying (http://www.compassionindying.org/) A pro-euthanasia organization designed to help those who want information to help them die. Several pro-euthanasia, pro-suicide articles.

Ethics Updates: Euthanasia (http://ethics.acusd.edu/euthanasia.html) Another great site from "Ethics Updates." A long list of resources including court cases, links, and lists of full text online articles. Go here first.

Euthanasia.com (http://www.euthanasia.com/) Literally tons of full text online articles dealing with different aspects of euthanasia issues.

Euthanasia Research & Guidance Organization (http://www.islandnet.com/~deathnet/ergo.html) Pro-euthanasia organization with many resources and links.

"Euthanasia: The Debate Continues" (http://www.mala.bc.ca/www/ipp/euthanas.htm) Good article that debates both sides of the issue by Bob Lane and Richard Dunton.

International Anti-Euthanasia Home Page (http://www.iaetf.org/) Provides a lot of information against active euthanasia and physician-assisted suicide.

CHAPTER 4

Death with Dignity: Physician-Assisted Suicide

Death with Dignity: Physician-Assisted Suicide

Introduction
A. Is Suicide Ever Justified?
B. What Is Physician-Assisted Suicide?
    1. Introduction
    2. The Maverick Model
    3. The Anonymous Philanthropist Model
    4. The Caring Personal Physician Model
C. The Legal Status of Physician-Assisted Suicide
    1. Court Cases
        a. People v. Kevorkian
        b. Compassion in Dying v. State of Washington
        c. Quill v. Vacco
        d. Washington v. Glucksberg; Quill v. Vacco
    2. State Legislation
D. Moral Arguments for and against Physician-Assisted Suicide
    1. Moral Arguments for PAS
        a. Introduction
        b. The Obligation of Physicians
        c. The Regulation Argument
    2. Moral Arguments against PAS
        a. Taking Life without Cause Fundamentally Wrong
        b. Too Much Vagueness in Preemptive Decisions
        c. Pain Management Allows for Relief of Suffering
        d. Misunderstanding of Death with Dignity
        e. Failure to Understand Why God Allows Things to Happen

4

Diane couldn't believe what she was hearing on the other end of the phone. She let out an expletive. "Don't tell me that," she said, followed by another expletive. She had been in for a check-up; she had a rash and had been feeling a little tired. The last word she ever expected to hear was, "leukemia." But that was the word he said. After all she had been through in her life. After conquering vaginal cancer, getting control over her alcoholism and depression and now — this.

Dr. Timothy Quill told her that he would run the blood count again, but he knew it would not change. It didn't. He called her and had her come into the hospital for more tests, including a bone marrow biopsy. In the end the tests confirmed what all hoped would not be true: Diane was suffering from acute myelomonocytic leukemia. Without treatment she had weeks, maybe a couple of months. With treatment Diane had about a 25% chance of long-term survival. However, treatment would not be easy. It involved a series of chemoterapy treatments followed by a bone marrow transplant. Because of her advanced stage the oncologist began to make plans for chemotherapy treatment to begin that afternoon. Diane became angry that he would presume that she wanted treatment. After agreeing to meet with Dr. Quill in two days, she went home.

Diane was a strong, independent, artistic woman. She was married and had a college-age son. They now sat in Dr. Quill's office two days later. Diane informed Dr. Quill that she had decided not to undergo the chemotherapy treatments, nor the bone marrow transplant. She had decided that the 25% chance was not high enough to go through the pain of treatment and loss of control that living in a hospital would force upon her in what were, most likely, her last days alive. Dr. Quill felt he could not disagree with her. Her family wished she would have chosen treatment, but had resigned themselves to her decision.

Dr. Quill and Diane met several times over the following week, and he was half expecting her to change her mind. He suggested that she consider hospice care when she grew closer to the time the disease would take over. However, Diane had a different idea. It was important for her to retain control and dignity and she was unsure she would be able to do so in a hospice care setting. She decided that, when the time came, she wanted to take her own life. Dr. Quill was reluctant to provide her with any support at first, thinking it was out of the realm of current medical practice. However, as he considered the possibility that she might do something violent, which would have terrible effects on the family, or that she might be unsuccessful and end up in a worse state, he informed her to contact the Hemlock Society. The Hemlock Society is an organization dedicated to helping those who want to painlessly end their lives.

Diane called back a week later requesting a prescription for barbiturates. Dr. Quill knew that overdosing barbiturates was a favorite suicide method of the Hemlock Society and he asked Diane to come into the office. Diane claimed that she had been experiencing insomnia, though Dr. Quill knew that she was only trying to protect him from possible legal impropriety. They spoke for a while and Dr. Quill became convinced that she was not acting out of depression or despondency. He wrote out a prescription for the pills and informed her of the correct dosage for insomnia as well as the amount needed to commit suicide. They agreed to continue meeting regularly and that she would see him before taking her life.

Over the next three months Diane went through good days and bad days. At one point it even looked like she was in remission. However, she suddenly began to decline very rapidly and it looked like the end was coming soon. The days Diane feared most were upon her — days of pain and dependence that could only be comforted by heavy sedation. She knew the time had come. She had friends stop by to say good-bye. She met with Dr. Quill and assured him she knew what she was doing. They tearfully said goodbye.

Two days later her husband called and said Diane was dead. She had said good-bye to her husband and son and asked to be left alone for about an hour. When they returned to the room she was lying on the couch with a shawl over herself. Dr. Quill came by and checked her then called the medical examiner's office. When asked the cause of death, he said she had died of acute leukemia. He justified his lie by claiming that he did not want an ambulance crew to arrive too soon and try to revive her, or for the family to suffer through an autopsy investigation. He was also concerned for the legal ramifications on the family and himself. However, Dr. Quill was bothered that Diane had to die alone and that he had to keep the real cause of her death a secret. He wondered how many other doctors and families had been involved in similar cases. And so, Dr. Quill decided to take Diane's story and publish it in one of the most prestigious medical journals in the country, *The New England Journal of Medicine*. When that issue hit the stands in 1991, it opened up a whole new debate in medical ethics.[1]

One's view of physician-assisted suicide (hereafter referred to as PAS) is obviously going to be affected by one's view of suicide itself. If one believes that suicide in general is unjustified, then it would seen difficult to justify physician-assisted suicide. I am not saying that it follows necessarily, but it would be inconsistent for one to reject suicide in a normative sense, and yet support PAS. Therefore it is necessary that we begin our study by answering the basic question first.

Is Suicide Ever Justified?

> *One's view of PAS is obviously going to be affected by one's view of suicide itself.*

What is suicide? One can define it in one of two ways. In a broad sense it is the intentional taking or forfeiting of one's own life. The problem with the broad definition of suicide is that it includes actions that most would not consider suicide in the traditional understanding of the term. For example, what of a person who knowingly and intentionally sacrifices his life for others, such as the soldier who throws himself on a grenade to save the life of his buddies? Few of us would call this a suicide. Or what of a Christian who refuses to recant his faith knowing that he will die if he does not agree to do so, yet he intentionally accepts death over recanting? This too would not be counted as a suicide by most persons. I would also suggest that refusal of treatment is not necessarily a suicide. It is possible that a patient may refuse treatment, even knowing such a refusal may end up in death, and yet he does not intend it. For example, Jehovah's Witnesses will usually refuse a blood transfusion due to religious beliefs and do so knowing that it may very well result in death. However, this does not mean that they are intending to die. In fact most hope that other methods of treatment can be used to save their lives. In short, we recognize that the broad definition of suicide is not appropriate due to many situations that are not usually considered suicide.

It is important to remember that a moral action is more than just intentions and actions — there is also the issue of motive. Whereas my intention describes *what* I am aiming for, my motive is a description of *why* I am aiming for it. To illustrate the difference, suppose a wealthy man is drowning and two men dive in with the intention of saving him. Even though they both have the same intention, to save the man, they may have totally different motives. One person may be the lifelong friend of this man and be saving him out of loyalty and love for their friendship. The other may be thinking that by saving this man he will get a financial reward. While we would admire both for doing the right thing, most of us would think lower of the man who did it for a *self-serving* motive over the one who did it for an *other-serving* motive. While self-serving actions are not always wrong (after all we do them all the time), it seems to most of us that there is rarely anything morally praiseworthy about them. We praise others when they put self aside for the sake of others.

What makes suicide different is motive.

I would like to suggest that what makes suicide different from other forms of intentional taking or forfeiting of one's life has to do with motive. A suicide is done for primarily self-serving motives as opposed to self-sacrifice which is primarily other regarding. Therefore I define a suicide as *the intentional taking or forfeiting one's life primarily for self-serving motives.* Does this definition answer every possibility or distinction between suicide and other actions? Perhaps not, but I believe it is a good working definition, and may be as good as we can get.[2] Philosopher Tom Beauchamp writes that it is "difficult to capture precisely which intention is required for suicide, and what the right excluding conditions are. Suicide is an ill-order concept, and the linguistic intuitions of indigenous users of the language are inadequate to correct it."[3]

Now that we have defined suicide, the question regarding its justification can now be addressed. In recent years several people have argued that suicide is a justifiable option in certain situations. Some of the main people who argue in favor of justified suicide are Derek Humphry, the founder of the Hemlock Society, Dr. Jack Kevorkian, and Dr. Timothy Quill. They have offered a number of arguments to support that view. First, the principle of respect for autonomy requires that people be allowed to commit suicide if they freely choose to do so. People have a right to privacy and a right to choose what to do with their own bodies. They have a right to choose when and how to die. Some have argued that this right is just as fundamental as the right to life. Second, rational suicide is possible. It is possible for a person to make a reasoned decision to end their life. The following criteria are usually advanced for a suicide to be deemed rational:(1) the immediate ability to reason, (2) a realistic worldview, (3) adequate information concerning his condition and its prognosis, (4) the desire to avoid harm or hurt to himself and others, and (5) the suicide is in accordance with his fundamental interests. Third, while it is true that human life has value, it is a relative value not an absolute one. It is possible to encounter a threshold where life has lost almost all its value. Those suffering in extreme pain and discomfort with little chance of recovery of the normal functions of human living would be an example. To require that these people maintain their lives is to condemn them to a life of agony. It would be more merciful to allow them to end their suffering and die with dignity.

How might one respond to these arguments? We have already commented about the autonomy issue in the last chapter and much of what we said there will apply here. First, it is an excessively individualistic concept of autonomy that argues it is "my life" without considering that one is a member of a community and has responsibilities to that community. Second, as Christians, we recognize that it simply isn't *your* life to do with as you please. We have a stewardship of responsibility to God for the life he has given to us. However, the one problem that comes out very strongly in the above arguments is that the first and second reasons counter each other. If it is my right to choose, then how can you place any conditions on it? The problem is that those who support suicide almost always support it under only certain conditions. For example, Derek Humphry writes: "We do not encourage any form of suicide for mental health or emotional reasons."[4] He then lists two justifying reasons for suicide: terminal illness in which suffering is present, and a grave handicap which is intolerable for the individual. He also lists at least seven "parameters" for justified suicide. However, if the main argument for justifiable suicide is respect for autonomy, why do I need any conditions or "parameters"? More importantly, since it is totally an individual choice, who are *you* to tell me what those conditions are?

> *If it is my right to choose, then how can you place any conditions on it?*

As far as the possibility of rational suicide itself, I believe one can reason to the conclusion that suicide is a proper course of action. However, while rational suicide is possible, it doesn't mean it actually occurs or that it is the morally right thing to do. A person can take a very rational approach to committing a crime, such as robbing a bank. They may have very self-interested goals that in light of their worldview make robbing a bank a reasonable action. The fact that it is rational is not an argument that it is morally justifiable. Also some raise the question of how often persons really are free from the mental or emotional conditions in order to make an objective, "rational" decision about their own death. Dr. Herbert Hendin is a psychiatrist and recognized authority on suicide. He is concerned that many of the supposed "rational" suicides may have been patients who were not adequately diagnosed and treated for depression, mental illness, or properly counseled about fear of pain, loss of control, and other end-of-life concerns. He writes:

Patients do not know what to expect and cannot foresee how their conditions will unfold as they decline toward death. Facing this ignorance, they fill the vacuum with their fantasies and fears. When these fears are dealt with by a caring and knowledgeable physician, the request for death usually disappears. . . . Unfortunately depression itself is commonly underdiagnosed and often inadequately treated. Although most people who kill themsleves are under medical care at the time of death, their physicians often fail to recognize the symptoms of depressive illness or, even if they do, fail to give adequate treatment.[5]

We also dealt with the mercy argument in the previous chapter. We saw that much has been done to alleviate pain in the area of medicines, technology and hospice care. Suicide supporters will often just refer to the autonomy argument and say that many just don't want to go that route. We have already discussed the problems with such a view of autonomy. Also we commented in the last chapter on communicating the wrong information about suffering. Lastly, the view that life only has a "relative" value and not "absolute" value is too subjective. Who becomes the determiner of life's value? Who decides where the "threshold" is? The only consistent answer is each individual himself. But then there is no regulation to suicide at all — it is totally up to each individual. The teenage girl who breaks up with a boyfriend and thinks life is no longer worth living has just as much of a "right to die" as the elderly person who has lost her husband and has no purpose in life. Humphry may assert that he would never encourage either of these situations, but such a strong view of autonomy insists that he must allow for them.

In opposition to the justifiable suicide view, is the traditional view of suicide. Traditionally throughout the majority of human history suicide has been viewed as an immoral act usually performed out of desperation, depression or mental illness. However, you find few actual arguments against suicide in older records. The reason is clear: arguments against suicide have only been recently advanced due to the fact that suicide has only recently been advocated as a justifiable act. No one bothered to argue against suicide because it was just assumed to be wrong. This is probably why there are no direct prohibitions against suicide in Scripture. There are five cases of suicide recorded in Scripture (Abimelech [Judg 9:54]; Saul [I Sam 31:4]; Zimri [I Kgs 16:18]; Ahithophel [II Sam 17:23]; Judas [Matt 27:5]) and all of them are in the context of God's judgment on shameful or sinful lives.

> *Traditionally suicide has been viewed as an immoral act.*

Those who argue for the traditional view usually offer the following arguments: (1) Suicide violates the fundamental principle of the sanctity of human life. All life has intrinsic value and one should never deliberately take or forfeit his own life without just cause. From a Christian point of view, life is a gift from God and we are created in the image of God. To take a life, even one's own, is to desecrate that image. (2) Suicide is contrary to the natural law. Humans have a natural human tendency to preserve their lives. It is natural for humans to live and to engage in human activities. Suicide perverts and violates this natural tendency. (3) Suicide harms society. It is an injury to family and friends and deprives society of an individual's contribution to it. By justifying suicide we condone its usage throughout all society. (4) Because reasons for suicide are subjective to each individual, there could be no objective way of regulating it.

What Is Physician-Assisted Suicide?

In answer to this question, we need to distinguish PAS from voluntary active euthanasia. They have much in common — so much that Tom Beauchamp places PAS as a subcategory of active euthanasia. They both involve the intentional death of a person, usually at his/her own request, and they both involve a third party. Also many of the arguments and problems we discussed under euthanasia will be applicable here. There are three distinctions that are important enough to warrant a separate look at PAS apart from euthanasia. First, PAS is specifically suggesting that a physician be involved in a patient's death, so there is the question of this being the proper role of a physician. Active euthanasia can be performed by anyone on anyone. Second, in PAS the physician is not the one who is actually administering the death-causing substance to the patient; the patient is administering it to himself. The physician is assisting in the person's suicide; he is not himself killing the patient. The moral relevance of this distinction is debatable, but it is a distinction. Third, active euthanasia almost always involves patients who are in the end stages of the dying process and are currently suffering. Assisted suicide may occur much earlier than the end stages of dying and, in several cases, the person has not been dying at all. While there is often some overlap between PAS and active euthanasia, these distinctions are enough to raise some important issues, though we shall see that many objections to active euthanasia will also be true of PAS. PAS can be defined as the intentional assistance of a physician in helping a patient to end his life through the provision of information and/or means necessary for them to accomplish that goal.

There are actually a number of different models of PAS. We will discuss three:

1. *The Maverick Model.* This model is best represented by Dr. Jack Kevorkian. Kevorkian is a pathologist living in Michigan. Beginning in 1990 he began to offer his services to those who wished to commit suicide. His first suicide "client" was Janet Adkins, a woman in the early stages of Alzheimer's disease. At the time Michigan had no law against assisted suicide and even after Kevorkian was admonished by the court not to repeat the incident, he continued to do so. In fact he makes a point of flouting any law or court request. He has helped more then 120 persons commit suicide in places ranging from their own homes to the back of his VW van. His normal method has been to attach them to a "suicide machine" that will first inject a saline solution, then a seda-

tive to put the person under, and finally potassium chloride which kills them. Until recently, Kevorkian himself did not perform the injection. The person committing the suicide pushed the button starting the machine. However, in a November 1998 broadcast of the news program *60 Minutes,* Kevorkian was seen injecting the patient himself, thereby moving from assisted suicide to active euthanasia. He was later arrested and, at the time of this writing, is awaiting trial.

Kevorkian's methods are considered crude even by proponents of PAS.

Kevorkian has come under criticism by both supporters and objectors of physician-assisted suicide for a number of reasons. His methods are considered crude, assisting suicides in the back of a van and then dumping bodies off at hospitals. Many are bothered that he is not the personal physician of any of his "patients," but appears on the scene just to help them die. In fact, he advocates a new medical discipline which he calls "obitiatry" — a medical specialty for physicians who just want to practice "medicide" — the killing of patients. The fact that he is not the regular personal physician of his "patients" means that he often hardly knows the people he is helping to die, often having just brief conversations with them before agreeing to help them die. He is not a clinical physician at all, but a pathologist. Many of his assisted suicides have been called into question. Herbert Hendin writes,

> In some of Kevorkian's cases the push for the patient's death came from relatives, in others no medical pathology was found on autopsy, and in virtually no case were any alternatives to assisted suicide adequately explored.[6]

Hendin goes on to report a number of questionable cases where Kevorkian has helped in suicides: people who, upon autopsy, were found not to be really sick, though Kevorkian insisted they were; people in suspicious situations, like when a husband arrested just three weeks earlier on a spousal assault charge helped arrange his wife's suicide; people of whom it is reported that they had doubts but felt pressured to go through with the suicide. Kevorkian does little of psychiatric investigation of the patients to see if they are suffering from depression or other abnormalities. He has employed a psychiatrist, Dr. George Reding, on occasion who briefly meets with patients, and admits to having apologized to them for having to subject them to a psychiatric examination. Reding himself admits to having practiced active euthanasia several times during his medical internship. Finally, Kevorkian seems to have a minimalist criteria for helping patients. He will help, not only those presently suffering, but people with "intense anxiety or psychic torture inflicted by self or others."[7] This virtually opens the door to anything Kevorkian wants to put in these categories. Kevorkian's license to practice medicine was suspended and he has been shunned by much of the medical community. His response is, "The medical profession made a mistake when they ostracized me. I have no career anymore. This is the substitute."[8] For these reasons, most people who argue for PAS are not arguing for the Maverick model.

2. *The Anonymous Philanthropist Model.* A controversial article appeared in the January 1988 issue of the *Journal of the American Medical Association* entitled "It's Over, Debbie." It relates the story by an anonymous resident being called late one night to the bedside of a 20-year-old woman dying of ovarian cancer. The physician had never met the woman and only knew her by her first name, Debbie. After spending some time attempting to comfort her pain, she made the ambiguous statement "Let's get this over with." With that the resident gave her an injection and she died quickly afterwards. This article was very controversial at the time, and both the physician as well as *JAMA* were heavily criticized for publishing it. Most critics, among whom were many supporters of physician-assisted suicide, believed that the resident acted wrongly in that he had inadequate knowledge of the patient

and the patient's illness to have taken action on such a vague request. This would also be considered more of a case of active euthanasia than assisted suicide. Most who are arguing for assisted suicide are not arguing for the anonymous philanthropist model.

Most who are arguing for assisted suicide are not arguing for the anonymous philanthropist model.

3. *The Caring Personal Physician Model.* More often cited as a good example of physician-assisted suicide is the case of Diane we related in the beginning of this chapter. This case first appeared as an article in the March 7, 1991, issue of *The New England Journal of Medicine* by Dr. Timothy Quill entitled "Death with Dignity: A Case of Individualized Decision Making." This example is the one often promoted as the type of physician-assisted suicide which should be legalized. The personal physician, who knows the patient and the patient's illness is involved. He provides the method for the suicide but leaves the ultimate decision in the patient's hands. Advocates argue that the shame in this case is that the woman had to do it alone and the doctor was forced to lie about the real cause of death. They would change those aspects if it were legalized.

Since publishing his case, Dr. Quill has published a number of articles and books advocating the legalization of PAS. In many of these he sets up a number of safeguards to assure that abuses do not occur. His proposed criteria include:

1. The patient must, of his own free will and at his own initiative, clearly and repeatedly request to die rather than continue suffering.

2. The patient's judgment must not be distorted — expert psychiatric evaluation should be sought if the primary physician is inexperienced in diagnosing depression.

3. The patient must have a condition that is incurable and associated with severe, unrelenting, intolerable suffering.

4. The physician must ensure that the patient's suffering and the request are not the result of inadequate comfort care.

5. Physician-assisted suicide should be carried out only in the context of a meaningful doctor-patient relationship.

6. Consultation with another experienced physician is required.

7. Clear documentation to support each condition above is required.[9]

Many advocates of PAS are favorably impressed with Dr. Quill's criteria. Other criteria have been suggested as well. Perhaps one of the most convoluted sets of criteria comes from the assisted suicide/voluntary euthanasia law for the Northern Territory of Australia which went into effect on July 1, 1996. It lists no less then 22 separate steps a patient must go through in order to obtain help from a physician in ending his or her own life. This law was overturned on March 25, 1997. It is models like these that are today being advocated as the type of PAS that should be legalized. Which brings us to the next issue.

The Legal Status of Physician-Assisted Suicide

Until recently the topics of assisted suicide and active euthanasia were largely confined to academic discussions and professional journals. However, events like the Kevorkian suicides along with the publication of articles like "It's Over, Debbie" and the case of Diane brought the topic more into the public square. In the 1990s there have been a number of movements to legalize assisted suicide, and some important cases have been argued in court. We will look first at the important cases before looking at the legislative activity.

Court Cases

1. *People v. Kevorkian* (1994). In the early 1990s a number of states began passing laws specifically outlawing assisted suicide. One of the most well known of these was the Michigan law, Public Act 270, which went into effect in February 1993 making it a felony to assist in a suicide, punishable by up to four years in prison. The law was a temporary ban that was written as a direct response to the assisted suicides performed

by Dr. Jack Kevorkian. After the act went into effect, Kevorkian assisted a terminally ill person in committing suicide in direct disobedience of the new law. Kevorkian was charged in district court for having violated the statute, and he moved to dismiss the charges claiming the law was unconstitutional: a person has a due process right to commit suicide, and the law places an undue burden on that right. The circuit court agreed and invalidated the statute. The case was appealed to the Michigan Court of Appeals which upheld the ruling of the lower court. The case was again appealed to the Michigan Supreme Court which ruled in May 1994 that the assisted suicide law did not violate the Michigan Constitution and therefore was a valid law. Kevorkian filed an appeal to the United States Supreme Court who refused to hear the case. The Michigan Supreme Court's ruling held. In November 1995 the temporary ban on assisted suicide expired, but the Michigan Supreme Court had ruled that assisted suicide is a felony under common law. In September 1998 the Governor signed into law a permanent ban on assisted suicide making it a felony.

To date Jack Kevorkian has been on trial four times for assisting in suicides. He has been acquitted three of those times by juries who believed he was not killing patients but relieving them of suffering. A fourth trial lasted one day and was declared a mistrial after Kevorkian's lawyer claimed that the prosecution had tampered with the evidence. At the time of this writing, Kevorkian is currently awaiting his fifth trial which will be under the new Michigan law.

2. *Compassion in Dying v. State of Washington* (1995, 1996). Washington state had a 146-year-old statute on the books stating that promoting a suicide by aiding or causing someone to commit suicide was a class C felony. In 1994 this law was challenged by a nonprofit organization called Compassion in Dying whose purpose was to help terminally ill persons to hasten their deaths. They challenged the constitutionality of the law claiming that it violated the due process clause of the Fourteenth Amendment of the U.S. Constitution. In May 1994, Judge Barbara Rothstein ruled in Federal District Court

for the Western District of Washington that the U.S. Constitution guaranteed a right to assisted suicide and that the statute was unconstitutional. The case was appealed to the Ninth Circuit Court of Appeals (49 F. 3d 586, 1995) where Judge Rothstein's decision was reversed. Judge John T. Noonan, highly regarded as one of the greatest legal minds in the country, wrote the majority opinion. Noonan held that there is nothing in the Constitution or in judicial precedents that supports the idea of a guaranteed "right to die." In fact he argues that legal judgments have ruled just the opposite. He writes that "A federal court should not invent a constitutional right unknown in the past and antithetical to the defense of human life that has been a chief responsibility of our constitutional government."[10]

> *Noonan held that there is nothing to support the idea of a guaranteed "right to die."*

A year later the case was appealed *en blanc* to an 11-judge panel in the Ninth Circuit (79 F.3d 790, 1996). The panel of judges reversed the Circuit Court of Appeals ruling. Judge Stephen Rinehart wrote the majority opinion. Rinehart claims that the 1993 *Casey* decision affirmed that "the heart of liberty is the right to define one's own concept of existence, of meaning, of the universe, and of the mystery of life." He held that this liberty, found within the Fourteenth Amendment, encompassed a right to determine the time and manner of one's own death. Rinehart also held that the distinction between killing and letting die was a distinction without a difference. Therefore he upheld the district court's original ruling that the Washington law was unconstitutional.

3. *Quill v. Vacco* (1996). In July 1994 a group of three physicians headed by Dr. Timothy Quill filed a complaint against the State of New York charging that the state laws prohibiting assisted suicide were unconstitutional, basing

their reasoning on the due process and equal protection clauses of the Fourteenth Amendment. The district court rejected the challenge, and it was appealed to the Second Circuit Court of Appeals. The Circuit Court announced its opinion on April 2, 1996, just a few weeks after the second *Compassion in Dying v. Washington* court announced its findings. Judge Miner, who wrote the court's opinion, rejected Rinehart's view that *Casey* supports a right to die, but ruled the New York laws unconstitutional on different grounds. Therefore, the New York laws prohibiting assisted suicide do not violate the due process clause. However, he did think they violated the equal protection clause. He ruled that the laws did not provide a rational basis for a distinction between terminally ill patients who chose to die by refusing treatment and those who chose to die through assisted suicide. This allowed for an unlawful discrimination against competent persons in the final stages of death who wished to hasten their deaths. Therefore the laws prohibiting assisted suicide were struck down.

4. *Washington v. Glucksberg; Quill v. Vacco* (1997). Both the Washington and New York cases were appealed to the United States Supreme Court. The court announced its ruling on both cases on June 26, 1997. In a unanimous ruling, it reversed the decisions of both the Ninth and Second Circuit Courts, ruling that states had a right to prohibit assisted suicide. Concerning *Washington v. Glucksberg*, Chief Justice Rehnquist stated that no precedent existed in American laws or custom that guaranteed a constitutional "right" to assisted suicide and, in a manner similar to Judge Noonan, stated that courts cannot create such a right from an abstract concept of personal autonomy. Therefore Washington's law does not violate due process as defined in the Constitution. Concerning the *Vacco v. Quill* case, Rehnquist argued that New York had a long history of distinguishing between killing and allowing someone to die which was widely recognized and rationally grounded. Therefore, the New York laws did not violate the equal protection clause as defined in the Constitution. Because

neither state's law prohibiting assisted suicide was found unconstitutional, they were allowed to stand. While these rulings were unanimous, five of the justices acknowledged the possibility that future laws prohibiting assisted suicide might be found unconstitutional.

Rehnquist stated that no precedent existed guaranteeing a "right" to assisted suicide.

In the last few years, five attempts have been made to legalize physician-assisted suicide. California has tried to legalize it twice. The first attempt (1988) did not even make it to the polls but fell short of getting the required number of signatures necessary to be placed on the ballot.

State Legislation

The second attempt occurred in 1992. It was called Proposition 161, The California Death with Dignity Act. It made it to the polls, but failed to gather a majority and was defeated 54%-46%. The year before California's second attempt, there was an attempt to legalize assisted suicide in the State of Washington. Called Initiative 119, the Washington Death with Dignity Act (1991), it proposed to permit doctors to lethally inject patients under certain circumstances. It was defeated in Washington by the same percentages as California: 54%-46%. It is because of this defeat in Washington that there was a change in tactics there and instead of passing a law legalizing assisted suicide, supporters decided to attempt to decriminalize assisted suicide and thus we had the Compassion in Dying cases discussed above. It is believed that both the Washington and California proposals were defeated because they were too broad and had few safeguards built in. This is a tactic that would soon change.

Before discussing the Oregon initiative in 1994, let us skip ahead to the most recent initiative, that is in the state of Michigan (1998).

The initiative in Michigan was Proposal B and was sponsored by Merian's Friends — a group named after a suicide patient of Kevorkian's, though the group claims to have nothing to do with Kevorkian himself and attempts to distance themselves from him. Proposal B was a 12,000 word proposal to legalize PAS. It had a large amount of safeguards built in to allay any fears concerning abuses. Kevorkian himself was actually against the proposal because he thought it would be too restrictive. However, even with the built-in safeguards, the proposal was soundly defeated 67%-33%. Critics charge that a massive campaign from the conservative right, full of misleading statements, was to blame for the defeat, though it seems that the margin of defeat is too great to be accounted for purely by misleading advertising.

In 1994 Oregon had a proposition on the ballot known as Measure 16: The Oregon Death with Dignity Act. The forces that had pushed for euthanasia in California and Washington had learned their lesson and toned down this proposition quite a bit, There were many more safeguards built into the law. Conservative forces were still rejoicing in the victories in the previous states and were unprepared for the campaign in Oregon. On Election Day the proposition was adopted as law by a slim majority: 52%-48%. Oregon had the distinction of becoming the first, and currently only, place in the world where PAS had been legalized.[11]

Oregon had the distinction of becoming the first, and currently only, place in the world where PAS had been legalized.

The Oregon law has a number of safeguards and criteria that must be met before a person can receive the medical drugs necessary to commit suicide. The patient must make the request twice with at least 15 days between the two requests. The rest of the burden is placed upon the physician who must: (1) first make an initial determination of whether a patient has a terminal disease in which he has six months or less to live, is capable, and has made the request voluntarily;

(2) inform the patient of: his/her medical diagnosis, prognosis, potential risks associated with taking medication to be prescribed, probable result of taking medication to be prescribed, any feasible alternatives, including, but not limited to comfort care, hospice care, and pain control; (3) refer the patient to a consulting physician for medical confirmation of disease and the time frame and for a determination that the patient is capable and acting voluntarily; (4) refer the patient for counseling if appropriate (counseling is required only if depression or another mental condition causes "impaired judgment"); (5) request that the patient notify the next of kin; (6) inform the patient that he or she has the opportunity to rescind the request at any time and offer the patient an opportunity to rescind at the end of a required 15-day waiting period from the date of the initial request to the writing of the prescription; (7) verify immediately prior to writing the prescription that the patient is making an informed decision; (8) fulfill medical record documentation requirements; and (9) ensure that all appropriate steps are carried out in accordance with this act.[12] After all these conditions are met, physicians would then be allowed, though not compelled, to write the prescription. It would be up to the patient to take the drugs. Physicians are not allowed to inject patients with drugs or give them injections to self-administer. The medicine prescribed is to be taken orally. Derek Humphry, president of the Hemlock Society and a resident of Oregon, was disappointed that doctors were not allowed to give injections.

Immediately, Right-to-Life groups sued the State of Oregon.

Immediately after passage, Right-to-Life groups and the Catholic Church, led by Dr. Gary Lee, sued the State of Oregon, and the law's validity came into question. The lawsuit charged that the law is discriminatory to the disabled and terminally ill, in essence saying that they are less deserving of protection than others for their lives could be taken without due process. On August 3, 1995, Federal District Judge Michael Hogan struck down the law on the basis that it was unconstitutional. His decision was based on the equal protection clause in the 14th amendment which holds that states may not deprive any citizen of life without due process of law. Judge Hogan stated, "certain fundamental rights cannot be dispensed with by majority vote."[13] However, in 1997 Hogan was overturned by the Ninth Circuit Court of Appeals due to a technicality when one of the plaintiffs in the original suit was deemed to not have standing. The case was appealed to the U.S. Supreme Court who refused to hear it. Since that time the Oregon State Legislature decided to put the matter before the people again and introduced Measure 51 on the 1997 ballot which would have repealed Measure 16. However Measure 51 was defeated this time by a wider majority than passed the original Death with Dignity Act. In light of these events Judge Hogan decided to dismiss the lawsuit but left the door open for the possibility of another suit in the future. Oregon remains the only place in the world where PAS is completely legal.

The status in the rest of the country stands as follows (as of July 1998): Thirty-seven states plus the District of Columbia have specific statutes on the books criminalizing assisted suicide. Nine states do not have specific laws against assisted suicide, but it is criminalized under the state common law against murder. Four states have no law prohibiting assisted suicide and have abolished common law criminal language against assisted suicide. As stated previously, only one state has legalized assisted suicide under state statute.

Moral Arguments for and against PAS

Moral Arguments for PAS

The two main moral arguments for PAS and for its legalization are the mercy argument, that people who are suffering should be allowed to end their suffering, and the autonomy or self-determination argument, that a person should be able to determine his own time and manner of death. We have already discussed these arguments in the previous chapter and earlier in this chapter and little can be added here that has not already been stated. However, since we are discussing legalizing assisted suicide, a comment made in the last chapter about the relationship between these two arguments needs to be amplified, for they are always conjoined together by those who argue in favor of legalizing assisted suicide. In strongly conjoining them, a major problem develops between these two arguments. Daniel Callahan comments:

> Once the key premises of the arguments are accepted, there will remain no logical way in the future to: (1) deny euthanasia to anyone who requests it for whatever reason, terminal illness or not; or to (2) deny it to the suffering *in*competent, even if they do not request it.[14]

The point is that there is no *a priori* reason why these two arguments should be linked together. Yet when they are separated, there are enormous problems for the pro-PAS view. Take autonomy for example. If an adult has a right to assisted suicide based on self-determination, then why do they have to be suffering? By requiring suffering, you have placed a limit on my self-determination. How does one justify this arbitrary limitation on autonomy? When we remove the suffering limitation, anyone can insist on assisted suicide for any desires or motivations.

By requiring suffering, you have placed a limit on my self-determination.

On the other hand consider the problem of the mercy argument. What happens to a person who is suffering but is presently or permanently incapacitated and not competent to make a decision concerning suicide? If the person is suffering, it seems unfair and merciless to say that they must continue to suffer simply because they are incompetent. Are they less entitled to relief from suffering than the competent? Again Callahan comments:

Each [argument] has its own logic . . . . But in the nature of the case that logic, it seems evident, offers little resistance to denying any competent person the right to be killed, sick or not; and little resistance to killing the incompetent, so long as there is good reason to believe they are suffering. There is no principled reason to reject that logic, and no reason to think it could long remain suppressed by the expedient of arbitrary legal stipulations.[15]

Here is a key point. If it is judged that the incompetent have a right to assisted suicide, and equal treatment demands we make such a judgment, then we must allow not only assisted suicide but also nonvoluntary active euthanasia. For the incompetent do not have the ability to request assistance in committing suicide. It will have to be done for them. Thus, while there is a legitimate distinction between assisted suicide and active euthanasia, to legally allow one, you must legally allow the other. Nicholas Dixon says: "Those who defend physician-assisted suicide often seek to distinguish it from active euthanasia, but in fact, the two acts face the same objections. Both can lead to abuse, both implicate the physician in the death of a patient, and both violate whatever objections there are to killing."[16] In light of this the arguments below will often be against both assisted suicide and active euthanasia.

> *If it is judged that the incompetent have a right to assisted suicide, then we must allow also nonvoluntary active euthanasia.*

Having dealt with the mercy and autonomy arguments previously, we will look at two arguments that are unique to PAS (and to a certain extent active euthanasia).

1. *The Obligation of Physicians.* One argument is based on the obligation that physicians owe their patients. According to this argument physicians have an obligation to help patients overcome pain and suffering and not to abandon them in their time of need. Since patients are autonomous

concerning their right to choose to die, physicians should be allowed to respect their autonomy and to help patients accomplish their goal in the most painless way possible and to insure its success. To say to a patient that they may commit suicide "on their own" without a physician's help is to abandon the patient.

This argument is based on the strong tradition in medical care that a physician cannot abandon a patient in need. This is referred to as "continuity of care." For example, the American Medical Association Council on Ethical and Judicial Affairs Code of Ethics has a section entitled "Fundamental Elements of the Patient-Physician Relationship." In that document they state that:

> The physician may not discontinue treatment of a patient as long as further treatment is medically indicated, without giving the patient reasonable assistance and sufficient opportunity to make alternative arrangements for care.[17]

However, there are a number of problems with this argument. First, the duty of a physician to not abandon a patient is a *prima facie* duty, meaning it upholds in most cases, but not necessarily all cases. For example, suppose a physician has a patient in need of a bone marrow transplant and he has found a compatible person to donate bone marrow, but the person refuses to participate. The physician's obligation to his patient does not allow him to force the person into donating against his or her will. In other words, one cannot justify doing anything one chooses based solely on the principle of loyalty to a patient. There may be situations when the duty to not abandon a patient may conflict with a more fundamental duty. Physicians also have a duty to do no harm and a duty not to kill. Many would argue that these duties of nonmaleficence are more fundamental than to provide continuity of care, which is a duty of beneficence.

Second, if the argument above is true, then physicians in fact really have no moral, and perhaps no legal, choice in the matter. They must honor their patient's wishes to be assisted in a suicide. But what if the physician believes that suicide is wrong? What if they think it is possibly justifiable in some cases, but not this one? His moral obligation of not abandoning his patient will not allow him to refuse to help him. The patient's autonomy ends up trumping the physician's autonomy. However, some PAS advocates will reply, "No physician will be forced to help a patient if that physician chooses not to. He may recommend the patient to a physician who will help the patient commit suicide." However, on what grounds could a doctor deny such a request? If it is true that his duty to honor self-determination and to relieve suffering are central to his profession, can he really deny a patient his "right" simply because of his "personal conscience"? As Callahan says, "The moral situation is radically changed once our self-determination *requires* the participation and assistance of a doctor."[18]

> *The patient's autonomy ends up trumping the physician's autonomy.*

Also, there are two problems with the PAS advocates' response. First, what if there are no other physicians who desire to assist in a suicide, or at least none within a reasonable proximity? This may place an "undue burden" on the patient, and it is possible the physician could be legally forced to honor the patient's wishes to carry out a treatment that has been deemed acceptable by law, but which the physician believes is wrong. Second, to pass the patient off to someone else is to ignore one of the main criteria of most advocates of PAS: Physician-assisted suicide should be carried out only in the context of a meaningful doctor-patient relationship. Behind this idea has always been the concept of a long-term relationship of the primary physician with the patient. However, what kind of meaningful relationship can be established by a physician and patient when that physician's only association with that patient is to help them die? This is more like the Maverick model of "obitiatrist" than the Quill model "caring physician."

A third problem has to do with what kind of judgment the physician is making here. The fact that the patient is requesting a medicinal method of committing suicide may lead one to believe this is medical decision. However, this is not a medical decision; it is a moral decision. Daniel Callahan brings this out in a discussion about euthanasia, but it applies also to assisted suicide:

> The doctor will not be able to use a medical standard. He or she will only be able to use a moral standard. Faced with a patient reporting great suffering, a doctor cannot, therefore justify euthanasia [or assisted suicide] on purely medical grounds (because suffering is unmeasurable and scientifically undiagnosable). To maintain professional and personal integrity, the doctor will have to justify it on his or her own moral grounds. The doctor must believe that a life of subjectively experienced intense suffering is not worth living. He must believe that himself if he is to be justified in taking the decisive and ultimate step of killing [or assisting in the killing of] the patient: it must be *his* moral reason to act, not the patient's.[19]

Assisting in suicide is not a medical decision;
it is a moral decision.

Again the problem is, what if the doctor holds the moral position that suicide is wrong? According to Callahan, he can't justify assisting someone on purely medical reasons, but he must justify them based on his own moral reasons. If he does not hold these moral reasons, then the abandonment argument says he must ignore his own conscience and fulfill his obligation to his patient. This obligation is even stronger if PAS is legalized or becomes an accepted standard of medical practice.

A fourth problem that many point out is that it is contrary to the traditional role of the physician as a health provider to now be in the business of hastening or helping in the death of patients. This tradition goes all the way back to the

Hippocratic oath which states in part, "I will apply dietetic measures for the benefit of the sick according to my ability and judgment; I will keep them from harm and injustice. *I will neither give a deadly drug to anybody if asked for it, nor will I make a suggestion to this effect.*"[20] Others have restated this basic principle of medical practice. A group of physicians, in responding to the "Debbie" case related above wrote:

> The resident violated one of the first and most hallowed canons of the medical ethic: doctors must not kill. Generations of physicians and commentators on medical ethics have under-scored and held fast to the distinction between ceasing useless treatments (or allowing to die) and active willful taking of life; at least since the Oath of Hippocrates, Western medicine has regarded the killing of patients, even on request, as a profound violation of the deepest meaning of the medical vocation. As recently as 1986, the Judicial Council of the American Medical Association, in an opinion regarding treatment of dying patients, affirmed the principle that a physician "should not intentionally cause death." Neither legal tolerance nor the best bedside manner can ever make killing medically ethical.[21]

What the sick need from the efforts of physicians is health.

David Orentlicher, an attorney for the AMA comments, "What the sick need and are entitled to seek from the efforts of physicians is health. Accordingly, physicians provide medical treatments to the sick to make them well, or as well as they can become. Treatment designed to bring on death, by definition, does not heal and is therefore fundamentally inconsistent with the physician's role in the patient-physician relationship."[22] Medical science simply cannot solve every problem. That is asking too much of it. The temptation to deal with one's frustration of not being able to solve every instance of suffering by ending life needs to be constantly checked. It is a Pandora's Box that we dare not open. If it is not checked, then medicine "becomes subservient to an undue aspiration for control: When the quality of *life* cannot be maintained at the desired level, the *situation* can be brought back under control by killing the patient."[23]

A fifth problem in requiring physicians to take on this new role, else they be guilty of abandoning their patients, is that there is good reason to believe that it will eventually undermine the physician-patient relationship. This can be illustrated by the cartoon of a man in bed who says to his wife, "I'm not feeling too well today, honey." His wife asks him if he would like her to call a doctor, to which the man replies, "I'm not THAT sick!" Even if the physician does not bring up the suicide option, it will be difficult for him not to influence the patient concerning it. Allowing the patient to act autonomously is giving him freedom to choose without substantial outside influence. Orentlicher points out why this is a problem in assisted suicide:

> *Even if the physician does not bring up the suicide option, it will be difficult for him not to influence the patient concerning it.*

If the physician appears sympathetic to the patient's interest in suicide, it may convey the impression that the physician feels the assisted suicide is a desirable alternative. Such an impression may not be very comforting to the patient. Moreover if the patient decides to reject suicide, will the patient have the same degree of confidence in the physician's commitment to his or her care as previously? In short assisted suicide might seriously undermine an essential element of the patient-physician relationship, the patient's trust that the physician is wholeheartedly devoted to caring for the patient's health.[24]

If the patient does not suggest assisted suicide, should the doctor bring it up as an option? As an aspect of informed consent, the physician is responsible to provide a list of all the viable options to a patient. If assisted suicide is legalized or becomes standard medical practice, the physician will be forced to offer it as an option. How would this affect a hopelessly ill patient? "He will not feel entirely free to resist a suggestion from the physician that suicide would be appropriate, particularly since it comes from the person whose medical judgment the patient relies on."[25]

2. *The Regulation Argument.* One of the major arguments raised against the legalization of PAS is that abuses are possible. People might be coerced into committing suicide, it might be extended to include those not terminally ill, etc. PAS advocates argue that while abuses are possible, criteria can be established that are effective projections against abuses by doctors and institutions. A number of suggested regulatory standards have been suggested including those above by Dr. Timothy Quill, the State of Oregon standards, and the "Model State" Standards provided by a group of Boston lawyers. Most of the regulatory standards have the same basic criteria: patient is competent in requesting it and repeats his request over time, severe pain or suffering with no other acceptable option in dealing with it, consultation with other doctors including a psychiatrist, good doctor-patient relationship, etc.

There are a number of problems with the concept of regulating PAS. Daniel Callahan and Margot White have written an excellent work dealing with many of these entitled "The Legalization of Physician-Assisted Suicide: Creating a Potemkin Village."[26] I will refer to some of the problems they raise. Some of these are general problems with the whole concept of regulation, while others are specific problems with criteria. First, those who argue for legislating PAS often say that assisted suicide is currently going on now in secret and that we need to legalize it so that it can be brought out in the public and properly controlled. The problem with this is that it admits that statutes probably won't help. If the present statutes outlawing PAS are ineffective in keeping people from abusing the law, what makes advocates think that regulation will be any more effective? If physicians don't take the law seriously now, what makes advocates think they will take it seriously later? They offer no evidence or studies to support the idea that regulation would really change any present practices. The vast majority of Kevorkian's suicides do not meet most of the regulatory criteria suggested by any of the advocates. Do they think that if it becomes legal, Kevorkian will stop his suicides? He has already said that the criteria suggested are too limiting. That gives us a hint of what he would do if PAS became legal — he would probably continue with what he is still doing. Probably so would most physicians who are currently breaking the law. There is no reason to believe regulating PAS would significantly help in any way.

*If the present statutes outlawing PAS
do not keep people from abusing the law,
how will regulation be any more effective?*

Second, even with all the regulation in effect the problem mentioned above of the power physicians have over patients, intentional or not, would render many regulations moot. While advocates argue that the final decision is with the patient, the physician can have an incredible influence over the patient. Callahan and White argue:

> As for the power of doctors, their general prestige as professionals whose training and experience are widely thought to enable them to understand matters of life and death better than the rest of us, and their capacity to give or withhold lethal drugs, already establish the power differential between them and their patients. . . the desire to medicalize PAS already bespeaks the power and legitimation conferred by medical approval of it.[27]

I am not implying that most physicians will abruptly and willingly force patients to accept suicide, though I think some might. But the majority who have accepted suicide as a legitimate way of dealing with a person can, even quite unknowingly, subtly pressure patients into committing the act. Herbert Hendin analyzes two examples of assisted suicide that advocates use to promote the right way it is to be done, and shows how the physicians pressured the patient, even while they were claiming several times that it was the patient's decision.[28]

In a videotaped case promoting PAS, a dying patient named Louise has requested suicide. Throughout the tape, the doctor, named Mero, and a member of Compassion for Dying are concerned that Louise might lose judgment before she goes through with the act. They are seen subtly pressuring her to commit suicide before it gets "too late." When Dr. Mero has to leave town for a while, he says "You don't need to wait for me." At another point Mero and a CFD member discuss how they can be more direct with Louise without actually telling her to hurry up (after all it has to be her idea). They say things to her and hope she will "read between the lines." While the doctor is out of town, Louise says she wants to wait until he is back before doing things. However, she is told, "Your doctor feels that if you don't do it this weekend, you may not be able to." At one point Louise blurts out, "I'm not afraid. *I just feel like everyone is ganging up on me.* I just want some time." Her mother then expresses concern that she will change her mind. Hendin, a trained psychiatric expert on suicide, tells us that, "Louise has expressed two conflicting wishes — to live and to die — and found support only for the latter. . . . Everyone — Mero, the friend, the mother, and the reporter — all became part of a network pressuring Louise to stick to her decision and to do so in a timely manner. The death was virtually clocked by their anxiety that she might want to live."[29] And this is an example of the way advocates think it should be!

A third problem with regulation is the issue of patient confidentiality. Medical decisions are made between a patient and physician in the privacy of the physician's office and with an agreement of confidentiality between them. If this practice is maintained, how is it going to be possible to monitor physicians to make sure they are remaining within the guidelines of the regulations? Callahan and White state: "We submit that maintaining the privacy of the physician-patient relationship and the confidentiality of these deliberations is *fundamentally incompatible* with meaningful oversight and adherence to any statutory regulations."[30] Again the fact that PAS is occurring today in secret demonstrates that it will continue in secret anytime it is not in keeping with the regulations.

As far as the specific regulations usually suggested, the concept of suffering presented in most of them is too vague and would eventually have to include those who are not terminally ill. Also the regulations either do not deal with the incompetent or those not physically able to commit suicide, or they must advocate active euthanasia (nonvoluntary for those who are incompetent) for them. Another problem with the suggested regulations has to do with the involvement of consulting physicians. The consulting physicians would have to be physicians who are already in favor of PAS in principle. Certainly physicians who are not in favor will not be involved in consulting on a PAS case. That would mean the thinking of the consulting physicians would be biased in favor of PAS, and therefore they might not be objective in judging a case. Callahan and White comment that often the regulations are set up more to *facilitate* PAS then to *regulate* it.

The best way to evaluate regulatory assisted suicide or euthanasia is to look at the Netherlands.

However, the best way to evaluate the success of regulatory assisted suicide or euthanasia is to look at a place where regulations have been in place for a while, the Netherlands. Before 1973 euthanasia was illegal and unacceptable in the Netherlands. In that year, a doctor was arrested and put on trial for killing her terminally ill mother with morphine. The court gave her a suspended sentence with one week in jail. This set a precedent, and courts quickly began to establish some guidelines on how to judge these kinds of cases. Euthanasia and assisted suicide were, and are, still illegal in the Netherlands and punishable by fine and imprisonment. However, physicians were immune from prosecution if they followed the court's basic guidelines. The basis for the immunity lies within the Dutch court's concept of *force majeure*. *Force majeure*, French for "superior force," is a legal term for an event or effect that cannot be reasonably anticipated or controlled. Hendin explains, "Euthanasia is thus permitted when a doctor faces an unresolvable conflict between the law, which makes euthanasia illegal, and his responsibility to help a patient whose irremediable suffering makes euthanasia necessary."[31] In 1984 the Royal Dutch Medical Association proposed a basic set of guidelines that standardized what the courts had been doing. The RDMA guidelines stipulate that euthanasia is excused if it is (1) voluntarily requested by a competent adult; (2) the request is based on full information; (3) the patient is in a situation of intolerable and hopeless suffering; (4) there are no acceptable alternatives to euthanasia; and (5) the physician has consulted another physician before performing euthanasia. Doctors were required to keep records of euthanasia cases and to report cases of euthanasia to the Dutch authorities. In 1994 the RDMA guidelines were made into government regulations by the Dutch Supreme Court.

How successful is the Dutch euthanasia program? In January 1990 the Dutch government appointed a commission to investigate the practice of euthanasia. It was headed up by Professor Jan Remmelink, attorney general for the Dutch supreme court. The commission interviewed 406 physicians and granted them anonymity and immunity from prosecution. The study was published in Dutch in 1991 and in English the following year. Its results were disturbing to many.

The Remmelink study found that 49,000 deaths in the Netherlands in 1990 involved a medical decision at the end of life.[32] Most of these deaths involved either the withholding or discontinuing of life support (passive euthanasia) or the alleviation of pain and symptoms through medication that might hasten death (i.e., a lethal dose was given with the intention to alleviate pain). However, 2,300 deaths were cases of active euthanasia (about 2% of all deaths in the Netherlands that year) and about 400 were assisted suicides. Most disturbing was the fact that just a little less than half of those euthanized, 1,040 of the 2,300, were actively killed *without the patient's knowledge or consent.* Of these 1,040, 14% were fully competent, 72% had never given any indication that they would want their lives terminated, and in 8% of the cases doctors performed involuntary euthanasia despite the fact that they believed alternative options were still possible. Forty-five percent of these nonvoluntary or involuntary euthanasia cases were performed without the consent or knowledge of the family. Over 50% of doctors admitted to practicing euthanasia. Only 60% kept a written record of their cases and only 29% filled out death certificates honestly, meaning that 71% of doctors did not report their involvement in euthanasia required by stated guidelines. All of these facts were infractions of the regulations then in place.

About 2% of all deaths in the Netherlands in 1990 were cases of active euthanasia, nearly half without the patient's knowledge or consent.

In addition to these 2,700 active euthanasia and PAS cases, the Remmelink report showed that 8,100 patients died as a result of doctors' deliberately giving them overdoses of pain medication, not for the primary purposes of controlling pain, but to hasten the patient's death. In 61% of these cases (4,941 patients) the intentional overdose was given *without the patient's consent.* In one report given to a 1990 bioethics conference in Maastricht, Holland, a physician from the Netherlands cancer institute told of approximately 30 cases a year where doctors ended patients' lives by first *intentionally* placing patients in a coma by means of morphine injections and then killing them. The physician said these were not considered euthanasia because they were not voluntary and to have discussed it with patients first would have been "rude" since they all knew they had incurable diseases.

Since the Remmelink report a landmark case occurred that extended euthanasia even more. The case concerned Dr. Boudewijn Chabot and a patient whom he calls Netty Boomsma. In July 1991 Dr. Chabot received a call from the Dutch Voluntary Euthanasia Society who referred him to a woman living in Assen who had lost both of her sons, one a few years earlier committed suicide and the other more recently died of cancer. Netty, who had left an abusive husband about three years earlier was depressed and had no one left in her life to care for. She did not believe there was any reason to live and desired to commit suicide. She specifically told Chabot that she did not want bereavement therapy. Chabot met with a number of experts and showed them his notes of Netty's case. Though most approved of the suicide, two of them advised him not to go through with it. One of these was the chair of the department of psychiatry at Erasmus University who believed that Netty needed therapy for her depression. Chabot asked only one of the experts to actually see Netty, and that expert declined, thinking it was not necessary. On September 27th Chabot met with Netty for the final time. He gave her some capsules, and she went upstairs, swallowed them, and died soon after. After Chabot reported that case, he was told he would have to appear in court. Netty was not terminal, she was not even dying, and she was not suffering in any physical sense. In other words it was a case of euthanasia that did not fall under the regulations. However, in April 1993 the court acquitted him and following two appeals, including one to the Dutch Supreme Court, he was exonerated. The court stated that mental suffering was grounds for suicide, though Chabot was chided for not having had a psychiatric consultant see her. This case is important because it establishes the precedent "that a patient a physician claims is not suffering from either psychiatric or physical illness can receive assisted suicide simply because he or she is unhappy."[33]

Two sad consequences come out of the Dutch euthanasia program. First, as Dr. Hendin testifies, rarely is adequate attention given to the mental state of patients who request suicide or euthanasia. Oftentimes psychiatrists are not called in at all to evaluate patients, or if they are called in, they only meet briefly with the patient and do not perform a full psychiatric evaluation or tests to see if the patient is suffering from clinical depression. In studying the cases over, Dr. Hendin is certain that the majority of them could have been helped with the right kind of therapy. However, because euthanasia and assisted suicide are readily available, it is just simply easier to immediately give in to the patient's desire and claim it was respect for self-determination rather than to help the patient through the difficult process of therapy.[34] The other sad consequence is that, according to a study of the British Medical Association, the state of palliative and hospice care in Holland is very poor.[35] Where euthanasia is an accepted medical solution to patients' pain and suffering, there is little incentive to develop programs which provide modern effective pain control for patients. As of the mid-1990s there were only two hospice programs in operation in the Netherlands.

It is just simply easier to immediately give in to the patient's desire and claim it was respect for self-determination rather than to help the patient through the difficult process of therapy.

It appears sufficient evidence from the Netherlands exists to call into question the whole idea of regulating assisted suicide as an assurance that abuses will not take place. Once we go down that avenue, there is no telling where we will end. The question is, if regulations have not stopped abuses from occurring in the Netherlands, what makes us think that we can stop them from occurring here?

Moral
Arguments
against PAS

Along with my criticisms of the moral arguments in favor of PAS, I wish to offer some arguments against it. First, it is fundamentally wrong to take human life without just cause. If a physician facilitates the taking of human life, then he is an accomplice to murder. Scripture is very clear about this. Exodus 20:13 gives the commandment not to kill; Jesus confirms this in Matthew 5:21; 19:18; Mark 10:19; and Luke 18:20. This command is based on the idea that man is made in the image of God and to kill man is to desecrate that image (Gen 9:6). Those who are suffering towards the ends of their lives are still image-of-God bearers. At no time does Scripture ever hint that these commandments are not in force even though many times people are suffering in Scripture. As mentioned earlier, though suicide is not specifically condemned, it is never condoned, can be considered self-murder, and in those places where people did commit suicide, it has a negative cloud hanging over it.

There is too much vagueness.

Second, there is too much vagueness in the area of preemptive decisions concerning suicide. **Preemptive suicide** is that which is undertaken not out of current suffering, but in anticipation of a predictably long, drawn-out decline in an illness. This is different from **surcease suicide**, that which is done as an escape from current suffering. In several of Kevorkian's assisted suicide cases the patients either were not terminal at all (Janet Adkins, Kevorkian's first suicide was in the very early stages of Alzheimer's disease with a prognosis of several years of alertness still ahead of her) or death was still quite far off. The vague question is how early should a person be allowed to be assisted in a suicide? One could push this to the absurd and argue that since we are all terminal, and more than likely will suffer from forms of deterioration throughout our life, that any of us could request assisted suicide now. To attach a time requirement of, for example, six months is simply to be arbitrary.

Third, in the cases of surcease suicides, recent techniques of pain management and the advent of hospice care have made it possible to treat virtually all pain and to relieve virtually all suffering. The dying process can be a valuable and positive experience of intimacy and spiritual growth. Rare instances of complete sedation can be used where pain cannot be controlled. While this is not the ideal situation, it is better then the taking of life and all of its ramifications.

Fourth, the concept of "death with dignity" is misunderstood by assisted-suicide advocates. To die with dignity is not so much an issue of the manner of your death (either immediately or drawn out) or the state you are in when you die (conscious or unconscious), but how you face death when it comes. It is recognition that death is a normal end to life and an acceptance of it as such. If anything, suicide has traditionally been seen not as death with dignity, but as a way to escape what life presents to you. A true death with dignity would respect life, see it as God's gift, and fight to keep it.

> *To die with dignity is more a case of how you face death when it comes.*

Finally, we cannot always answer the question of why God allows certain things to happen. But we have an obligation to live in faithfulness to him because this is not our life, it is his. Christian ethicist Stanley Hauerwas makes this point:

> The language of gift does not presuppose we have a "natural desire to live," but rather that our living is an obligation. It is an obligation that we at once owe our creator and one another. For our creaturely status is but a reminder that our existence is not secured by our own power, but rather requires the constant care of, and trust in, others. Our willingness to live in the face of suffering, pain, and sheer boredom of life is morally a service to one another as it is a sign that life can be

endured and moreover our living can be done with joy and exuberance. Our obligation to sustain our lives even when they are threatened with, or require living with, a horrible disease is our way of being faithful to the trust that has sustained us in health and now in illness. We take on a responsibility as sick people. That responsibility is simply to keep on living, as it is our way of gesturing to those who care for us that we can be trusted and trust them even in our illness.[36]

ENDNOTES

[1]The story is a summary of the story as it is told by Dr. Timothy Quill, "Death with Dignity: A Case of Individualized Decision Making"(1991), reprinted in *Last Rights: Assisted Suicide and Euthanasia Debated*, ed. by Michael M. Uhlmann (Grand Rapids: Eerdmans, 1998).

[2]For example, some might argue that a person who commits suicide so as not to be a financial burden to their family is acting in an other-regarding manner. However, I agree with J.P. Moreland, that this is not so much a regard for others themselves as it is a regard for others' nonpersonal states of affairs (i.e., their wealth). See J.P. Moreland, *The Life and Death Debate: Moral Issues of Our Time*, with Norman L. Geisler (Westport, CT: Greenwood Press, 1991), p. 87.

[3]Tom L. Beauchamp, "The Problem of Defining Suicide," in *Ethical Issues in Death and Dying*, 2nd ed., ed. by Tom L. Beauchamp and Robert M. Veatch (Upper Saddle River, NJ: Prentice-Hall, 1996), p. 117.

[4]Derek Humphry, "The Case for Rational Suicide," in *Last Rights*, p. 307.

[5]Herbert Hendin, M.D., *Seduced by Death: Doctors, Patients, and Assisted Suicide* (New York: W.W. Norton, 1998), pp. 34-36.

[6]Ibid., p. 43.

[7]Jack Kevorkian, *Prescription: Medicide: The Goodness of Planned Death* (Buffalo, NY: Prometheus Books, 1991), p. 318.

[8]Hendin, *Seduced*, p. 43.

[9]Dr. Timothy E. Quill, "Potential Criteria for Physician-Assisted Suicide" (1993), reprinted in Uhlmann, *Last Rights*, pp. 330-332.

[10] *Compassion in Dying v. State of Washington*, 49 F, 3d 586, March 9, 1995.

[11]As mentioned earlier, the Northern Territories of Australia was the first place to legalize voluntary euthanasia on July 1, 1996. However, that law was overturned on March 25, 1997. Contrary to some misunderstandings, PAS and euthanasia are not legal in the Netherlands. They are tolerated and not prosecuted.

[12]This summary of the conditions of the law is taken from Wesley J. Smith, *Forced Exit: The Slippery Slope from Assisted Suicide to Legalized Murder* (New York: Random House, 1997), pp. 121-122.

[13]*Lee v. State of Oregon*, 891 F. Supp., 1995.

[14]Daniel Callahan, "Physician-Assisted Suicide Should Not Be Legal" (1991), reprinted in *Suicide: Opposing Viewpoints* (San Diego: Greenhaven Press, 1992), p. 72, emphasis mine.

[15]Callahan, "Physician-Assisted Suicide," p. 73.

[16]Nicholas Dixon, "On the Difference between Physician-Assisted Suicide and Active Euthanasia," *Hastings Center Report*, 28:5 (Sept-Oct 1998), p. 25.

[17]AMACEJA, "Fundamental Elements of the Patient-Physician Relationship" (1994), reprinted in *Contemporary Issues in Bioethics*, 5th ed., ed. by Tom L. Beauchamp and LeRoy Walters (Belmont, CA: Wadsworth Publishing, 1999), p. 40.

[18]Callahan, "Physician-Assisted Suicide," p. 73. emphasis mine.

[19]Callahan, "Physician-Assisted Suicide," p. 73.

[20]Hippocratic Oath, 4th century, BC, reprinted in Beauchamp and Walters, p. 39, emphasis mine.

[21]Willard Gaylin, Leon R. Kass, Edmund R. Pellegrino, and Mark Siegler, "Doctors Must Not Kill" (1988), reprinted in *Arguing Euthanasia: The Controversy over Mercy Killing, Assisted Suicide, and the Right to Die*, ed. by Jonathan D. Moreno (New York: Simon and Schuster, 1995), p. 34.

[22]David Orentlicher, "Physicians Cannot Ethically Assist in Suicide" (1991), in Michael Biskup, *Suicide: Opposing Viewpoints*, p. 61.

[23]Henk Jochemsen, "The Netherlands Experiment," in *Dignity and Dying: A Christian Appraisal*, ed. by John F. Kilner, Arlene B. Miller, and Edmund D. Pelligrino (Grand Rapids: Eerdmans, 1996), p. 176.

[24]Orentlicher, "Physicians," p. 59.

[25]Ibid., 59-60, citing Yale Kamiser, source unknown.

[26]Potemkin Villages were fake villages erected in Russia in order to hide the slums from the Empress as she rode through the country.

[27]Daniel Callahan and Margot White, "The Legalization of Physician-Assisted Suicide: Creating a Potemkin Village," in Uhlmann, *Last Rights*, p. 580.

[28]Herbert Hendin, "Selling Death and Dignity," *Hastings Center Report*, 25:3 (May-June, 1995), pp. 19-23.

[29]Ibid., pp. 21-22.

[30]Callahan and White, "Legalization," p. 581.

[31]Hendin, *Seduced*, p. 64.

[32]*Medical Decisions about the End of Life*, The Hague, September 19, 1991. All of the following statistics come from the above report.

[33]Hendin, *Seduced*, p. 84.

[34]Hendin, *Seduced*, pp. 155-162.

[35]*Euthanasia: Report of the Working Party to Review the British Medical Association's Guidance on Euthanasia*, British Medical Association (May 5, 1988), p. 49.

[36]Stanley Hauerwas, *Suffering Presence: Theological Reflections on Medicine, the Mentally Handicapped, and the Church* (Notre Dame, IN: University of Notre Dame Press, 1986), p. 106.

References

Books on Suicide and Physician-Assisted Suicide

Battin, Margaret Pabst. *Ethical Issues in Suicide*. Englewood Cliffs, NJ: Prentice-Hall, 1995.

Battin, Margaret P., Rosamond Rhodes, and Anita Silvers. *Physician-Assisted Suicide: Expanding the Debate*. New York: Routledge, 1998.

Beauchamp, Tom L., ed. *Intending Death: The Ethics of Assisted Suicide and Euthanasia*. Upper Saddle River, NJ: Prentice-Hall, 1996.

Beauchamp, Tom L. and Robert M. Veatch. *Ethical Issues in Death and Dying*. 2nd ed. Upper Saddle River, NJ: Prentice-Hall, 1996.

Biskup, Michael. *Suicide: Opposing Viewpoints*. San Diego: Greenhaven Press, 1992.

Demy, Timothy J. and Gary P. Stewart. *Suicide: A Christian Response*. Grand Rapids: Kregel Publications, 1998.

Hamel, Ronald P. and Edwin R. DuBose. *Must We Suffer Our Way to Death? Cultural and Theological Perspectives on Death by Choice*. Dallas: Southern Methodist University Press, 1996.

Hendin, Herbert. *Seduced by Death: Doctors, Patients, and Assisted Suicide*. Boston: W.W. Norton, 1998.

Kilner, John F., Arlene B. Miller, and Edmund D. Pellegrino. *Dignity and Dying: A Christian Appraisal*. Grand Rapids: Eerdmans, 1996.

Moreland, J.P. and Norman L. Geisler. *The Life and Death Debate: Moral Issues of Our Time*. Westport, CT: Greenwood Press, 1990.

Moreno, Jonathan D. *Arguing Euthanasia*. New York: Touchstone (Simon and Schuster), 1995.

Smith, Wesley J. *Forced Exit: The Slippery Slope from Assisted Suicide to Legalized Murder*. New York: Random House, 1997.

Stewart, Gary P., et al. *Basic Questions on Suicide and Euthanasia: Are They Ever Right?* Grand Rapids: Kregel Publications, 1998.

Uhlmann, Michael M. ed. *Last Rights: Assisted Suicide and Euthanasia Debated*. Grand Rapids: Eerdmans, 1998.

Websites on Physician-Assisted Suicide: (See Chapter 3 for other sites relating to Physician-Assisted Suicide.)

Assisted-Suicide Information at Right to Life of Michigan (http://www.rtl.org/) A very good site for information especially dealing with Michigan's struggle with assisted suicide.

Euthanasia and Physician Assisted Suicide: All Sides (http://www.religious tolerance.org/euthanas.htm) A site that attempts to present all sorts of different sides to the euthanasia and assisted suicide debate.

Euthanasia.com (http://www.euthanasia.com/) Literally tons of full text online articles dealing with different aspects of euthanasia issues.

Hemlock Society USA (http://www2.privatei.com/hemlock/) A site that argues vigorously for assisted suicide by the premier suicide advocacy group in the country.

International Anti-Euthanasia Home Page (http://www.iaetf.org/) A lot of information against active euthanasia and physician-assisted suicide.

The Kevorkian File (http://www.rights.org/deathnet/KevorkianFile.html) A Pro-Kevorkian site.

The Kevorkian Papers(http://www.interlife.org/kevorkian/) Articles and information with a slant against Kevorkian.

Yahoo! Full Coverage — Assisted Suicide (http://headlines.yahoo.com/Full_Coverage/US/Assisted_Suicide/) A great site sponsored by Yahoo that keeps a running list of the most recent articles on physician-assisted suicide.

CHAPTER 5
From Cradle to Coffin: Imperiled Newborns

From Cradle to Coffin: Imperiled Newborns

5

Dan and Linda were eagerly awaiting the birth of their baby. They were a young couple who had only been married a short while when Linda became pregnant. Dan had worked hard expanding their small home in eastern Long Island and had built two extra rooms one of which would be a nursery. They were like any of a number of lower-middle-class couples just starting out in life. They never dreamed the birth of this baby would thrust them into the national spotlight.

Kerri-Lynn was born on the morning of October 11, 1983, at St. Charles Hospital on Long Island. She weighed 6 pounds and was 20 inches long. Immediately everyone could see that Kerri-Lynn was badly impaired. On her back was a protruding bubble-shaped membrane with the spine exposed. This is called a *meningocele,* and occurs when a gap does not close between two vertebrae in a developing fetus. This gap allows the *meninges,* a membrane that covers the spinal cord, to develop outside on the baby's back. Upon seeing the protrusion, the doctors knew that Kerri-Lynn was born with *spina bifida cystica.* If left untreated, Kerri-Lynn would likely die within a year or two. If treated, it would mean a lifetime of operations and severe physical handicaps.

Unfortunately, that was not Kerri-Lynn's only problem. She also had a damaged kidney and microcephaly. Microcephaly means that Kerri-Lynn was born with her head much smaller than normal, implying a minimal brain. This usually is a sign of mental retardation. On top of all this she had some of the usual disabilities that are found in *spina bifida* babies, including *hydrocephalus,* which is an abnormal accumulation of fluid on the brain. Kerri-Lynn was immediately transferred to the neonatal intensive care unit (NICU) at the University Hospital of the State University of New York campus at Stony Brook, Long Island. Two physicians, a surgeon named Arjen Keuskamp and a pediatric neurologist named George Newman, became involved in Kerri-Lynn's case. Controversy and disagreement started immediately. The issue was the problem of the hydrocephalus which needed to be drained immediately or Kerri-Lynn would become even more severely retarded or even die. Keuskamp recommended immediate surgery and draining of the hydrocephalus to minimize retardation and get the child out of the immediate danger of death. Newman disagreed and upon examining Kerri-Lynn consulted with Dan about midnight, 14 hours after Kerri-Lynn was born. Newman told Dan there were two options. They could perform the surgery that would save Kerri-Lynn's life. But that would likely leave her paralyzed, retarded and vulnerable to bladder and bowel infections for the rest of her life, and she probably would not live beyond her teenage years, if that long. Newman said, "She is not likely to achieve any meaningful interaction with her environment, nor ever achieve any interpersonal relationships, the very qualities which we consider human."[1] The other option would be to forgo the surgery and allow Kerri-Lynn to die soon, sparing her from such a life.

Dan and Linda went through the agony of having to make a terrible choice. After talking together and then with others, they decided not to have the operation and allow Kerri-Lynn to die. The baby went from being impaired to being imperiled. She received palliative care: food, water and antibiotics. Everyone assumed she would die in just a couple of days. However, four days later Kerri-Lynn was still alive. Kathleen Kerr, a reporter for *Newsday* magazine got wind of the story and interviewed the couple. It was important to Dan and Linda to express that their decision had been made out of love for Kerri-Lynn. Kerr's story broke on October 18, 1983, and with its publication came the winds of fury.

A History of Imperiled Newborns   The fact that having a baby is one of the greatest joys we can ever experience is what makes the tragedy of a congenital disease or other infant handicap so hard for most of us to accept. About 3.7 million babies are born per year in this country[2] and a significant number of them are born severely impaired. Some of the conditions are: heart malformations (~4,500), Down's syndrome (~1,600), spina bifida cystica (~ 1,000), **anencephaly** (~1,000), and extreme prematurity (~52,000).[3] Until recently, infants born in these conditions often had little chance of survival beyond a few years or, in some cases, days. However, with the advances in medical knowledge and procedures many of these cases have much better chances of survival. In 1950 the infant mortality rate in the country was 29.2 per 1,000 births. By 1996 it had dropped to 7.3 per 1,000 births. In 1950, 17.8 per 1,000 impaired newborns did not survive in neonatal units beyond 7 days. By 1996 the figure had dropped to 3.8 per 1,000. However, this new technology also raised some serious ethical questions: Who should make decisions about the care of these infants? Is it ever justified to cease or forgo treatment for impaired newborns? What would such nontreatment entail? Is active euthanasia ever justified in these situations?

Infanticide, the practice of allowing infants to die, or of killing infants, is not new. Throughout history many different cultures have practiced killing newborns for a variety of reasons: physical abnormalities, sex selection, economic considerations, and social considerations. Plato and Aristotle both advocated it in some situations. It was practiced later in Rome when children were simply abandoned in fields and left to die. Among the Bedouin tribes of Arabia, in China and in much of India firstborn female infants were often killed so that the firstborn would be a son. However, the religious traditions of the three great western religions — Islam, Judaism and Christianity — strongly condemned most cases of infanticide and affected many of the cultures in which they arose. In modern times most civilized cultures do not practice infanticide in any but the rarest situations. However, in recent years infanticide has entered the medical community and now a new term has developed — **neonaticide**. It would be helpful to see how this has developed.

The three great western religions strongly condemned most cases of infanticide.

In 1972 the Johns Hopkins Hospital in Baltimore, Maryland, released a film called *Who Should Survive?* It told the story of an infant boy who had been born the previous year with Down's syndrome. Down's syndrome, named after Langdon Down who discovered it, is a chromosomal abnormality in which a person has 47 chromosomes instead of the normal 46. The extra chromosome is on chromosome 21, and therefore the disease is technically called Trisomy 21. Trisomy 21 is a genetic condition that almost always causes some form of mental retardation (either mild or severe), facial abnormality (which is why it used to be called *mongolism*), and about a third of the cases are accompanied by cardiac or intestinal problems. Such was the case of a child born at Johns Hopkins.

The Down's syndrome baby had a duodenal atresia, or bowel obstruction. Without surgery, the natural flow and digestion of food could not take place and the child would die. The surgery to correct such a problem was relatively routine and on any normal child would have taken place without question. However, both parents, one a nurse who worked with Down's syndrome children and the other a lawyer, refused to consent to the surgery. Their reasons were never specifically stated, though the manner in which they spoke suggested they felt they either couldn't, or just didn't want to, care for a Down's syndrome child. The pediatric surgeons honored their wishes. The child was not fed intravenously and died of starvation and malnutrition 15 days later. The film documenting the case was shown throughout the country. As a result other doctors began to go public in the early 1970s. Duff and Campbell, two pediatricians at the Yale-New Haven Medical Center admitted to accepting parents' decisions to forgo treatment of 43 impaired infants who all died.[4]

The next significant event in the history of imperiled newborns occurred on May 5, 1981, when conjoined twins, Jeff and Scott, were born to Pamela and Robert Mueller in Danville, Illinois. They became known as the "Danville Twins." The twins were joined at the trunk and shared three legs. The Muellers decided they did not want any aggressive treatment and asked that the boys be allowed to die. However, Child Protection Services stepped in and obtained a court order for temporary custody of the children. The Muellers were charged with child neglect, but the charges were later dropped, and custody was returned to them in September 1981 when pediatric surgeons testified that a separation would not be successful and the prognosis for survival was very poor. The twins were eventually separated and as a result Scott died but Jeff survived.

The landmark case for imperiled newborns occurred in 1982.

The landmark case for imperiled newborns occurred in 1982. On April 9, 1982 a baby was born in Bloomington, Indiana, with Down's syndrome and suffering from tracheo-esophageal fistula. This was a small gap located in the area of the windpipe and esophagus preventing passage of food to the stomach. This condition could be corrected with surgery which is fairly standard and was given an 80%-90% chance of success. According to Pence, the obstetrician, Walter Owens, downplayed the chances of a successful operation and emphasized the tragedy of Down's syndrome, saying that these children are little more than "blobs" and that the lifetime cost of treatment would be close to a million dollars.[5] The parents decided not to operate based on their physician's prognosis and the baby's having Down's syndrome.

The hospital attempted to get a court order to operate and had an emergency meeting with a county judge, John Baker, late that night at the hospital. No official record of the meeting was made. The obstetrician again emphasized the poor condition of Down's syndrome children saying that even a minimum quality of life was nonexistent. The infant's father, who by this time had become convinced by the obstetrician, said he did not want the child treated. The judge ruled that the parents had the right to make the decision about treatment for their children. The case was appealed to the Circuit Court and to the Indiana State Supreme Court who both upheld the lower judge's ruling. While attempting to appeal to a U.S. Supreme Court Justice in order to get a stay, the baby died. This made the case moot.

On the basis of the media blitz concerning this case, the Reagan Administration directed the Justice Department and the Department of Health and Human Services to mandate that all hospitals which practiced this kind of infanticide, would lose all federal funding. This was based mostly on

Section 504 of the Rehabilitation Act of 1973, which forbade discrimination solely on the basis of handicap. The reasoning was that infants were citizens and it was a violation of their civil rights to end their life solely on the basis of being handicapped. The Justice department and HHS established a set of guidelines requiring treatment of all newborns regardless of handicaps. These became known as the **Baby Doe Laws**.

The original laws went into effect on March 21, 1983. Notices were sent to all hospitals concerning the laws and large posters were hung around NICUs informing all that it was against federal law to discriminate against handicapped newborns by not feeding or caring for them. A hotline number was set up to report any abuses. Teams of investigators were established, nicknamed "Baby Doe Squads." Many pediatricians became concerned that any crackpot could call the hotline and report them for almost any sort of a violation, making it impossible to work under such an oppressive environment. The American Association of Pediatrics filed suit in federal district court almost immediately after the laws went into effect. On April 14, 1983, the court decided in favor of the AAP and put a stop to the Baby Doe Laws. However, the suit was decided purely on a technicality and by February 12, 1984, new Baby Doe Laws were in place.

This brings us to the case of Kerri-Lynn, or Baby Jane Doe as she was referred to at the time. On October 18, 1983, the same day Kathleen Kerr published her interview with Dan and Linda, a Vermont lawyer named Lawrence Washburn filed suit in a Long Island courtroom on Kerri-Lynn's behalf to force treatment. On October 20th a lower court hearing was held, presided over by Judge Melvyn Tannenbaum. Because Washburn didn't have legal standing, the judge appointed a guardian *ad litem* ("for the case"), for Kerri-Lynn. He was a local lawyer, William Weber, who was empowered to make medical decisions for Kerri-Lynn. Weber was sympathetic to Dan and Linda and was going to move in favor of nontreatment until he read some comments that Newman, the pediatric neurologist, had written in Kerri-Lynn's chart. Newman, who had told Dan that Kerri-Lynn would be paralyzed, had written in the chart that after surgery, Kerri Lynn would probably be able to walk with braces. Obviously she would not necessarily be paralyzed as they had been led to believe. He also read that her head measured 31 centimeters, which was within normal limits and therefore Kerri-Lynn did not have microcephaly. On October 20 Weber authorized the surgery to take place.

Meanwhile the lawyer for Kerri-Lynn's parents, Paul Gianelli, appealed to the Appellate Division of the State Supreme Court. On October 21 they overturned Tannenbaum's original decision to appoint Weber as Kerri-Lynn's guardian. The court said the decision should be left to the parents when it is between two medically reasonable options. Weber appealed to the New York Court of Appeals. On October 28 the court announced its decision to uphold the parents' right to decide, stating that this should never have been brought to court as there was no neglect present and that Washburn and Weber should never have been involved.

> *The court said the decision should be left to the parents when it is between two medically reasonable options.*

By this time the case had gained national attention. Even before the New York Court of Appeals rendered its verdict, the federal government stepped in. On October 22 members of the "Baby Doe Squad" notified Stony Brook hospital to turn over Kerri-Lynn's medical records to see if she had been discriminated against according to Section 504 of the Rehabilitation Act. On October 25 the hospital announced that it would refuse to do so. On the 27th the HHS turned the case over to the Justice Department, who filed suit against the hospital in federal court on October 29. In late November the federal court ruled that the hospital did not need to release the records. The judge, Leonard Wexler, decided that the decision not to treat Kerri-Lynn was not discriminatory. The case was appealed to the Second Circuit Court of Appeals which, on February 23, 1984, agreed with the lower court and denied the government access to Kerri-Lynn's file.

In a last desperate move the Justice Department appealed to the United States Supreme Court. The case was argued before the court as *Bowen v. American Hospital Association* on January 15, 1986, and they rendered their decision in the case on June 9, 1986. The court held that (1) the records did not need to be released, (2) no evidence was present that Kerri-Lynn was subjected to discriminatory treatment, (3) the hospital was not guilty of any discrimination because it was the father who was denying treatment, not the hospital, and Section 504 didn't apply to the father, and (4) Section 504 of the Rehabilitative Act was never intended to be used as a club by the federal government to step in and mandate treatment decisions between hospitals and patients. With that decision the Baby Doe Laws were dealt the final blow.

Since the Baby Jane Doe case, there has been little attempt to prosecute parents who make nontreatment decisions.

Since the Baby Jane Doe case, there has been little in the way of attempting to prosecute parents in cases where they make nontreatment decisions, unless it is overwhelmingly obvious that treatment should have taken place and the hospital complied with the wishes of the parents — such cases are practically nonexistent. The feeling is that a jury won't convict a parent for nontreatment of a badly impaired newborn. The one case that has come up demonstrates this is true. In Chicago in 1989 Dan Linares held an entire NICU staff at gunpoint while he disconnected his 16-month-old son, Rudy, from a respirator. Rudy had been in a persistent vegetative state for nine months after choking on a balloon at a birthday party. Linares was charged with first-degree murder, but the grand jury refused to indict him for homicide.

In 1984 Congress amended the Child Abuse Prevention and Treatment Act of 1974 to count nontreatment of impaired newborns as medical neglect and therefore a form of child abuse and made individual states responsible for enforcement of the act. In 1992 the Americans with Disabilities Act went into effect and was applied to the "Baby K" case which we will discuss below.

What about Kerri-Lynn? Well at some point during all the different court appeals, Dan and Linda changed their minds and decided to have the operation to drain her hydrocephalus. She continued to live and was taken home on April 7, 1984, at five months. At this time a doctor predicted that she would be bedridden her entire life. However, in an article written by Kathleen Kerr six years later it was reported that Kerri-Lynn was seven years old and doing remarkably well. She was in a special education program and was rated between educable-retarded and low-normal. She was confined to a wheelchair and her speech was somewhat muddled, but she could talk. She still needed to be catheterized four times a day. Despite all the dire predictions, however, she was able to play with friends and was, generally a happy child.[6] As far as is known she is still alive today.

Despite all the dire predictions, Kerri-Lynn grew into a generally happy child.

There are two ethical questions we need to discuss concerning the nontreatment of imperiled newborns. First, who should decide in these cases? Second, on what basis should decisions to forgo treatment and allow infants to die be made? The first question will be addressed briefly and we will spend more time addressing the second.

Moral Arguments Concerning Imperiled Newborns

Who should decide about treatment in cases of severely impaired newborns? The first reply would obviously be the parents. After all, it is their child and they are the ones who are legally and morally responsible for its upbringing. Patricia Phillips writes:

> Since the family must live with the consequences of any decision made with regard to sustaining or withholding treatment, it is imperative that the decision ultimately is left to the parents. Neither physicians, hospital infant care review committees, nor the legal system should be permitted to usurp the fundamental right that abides in parents to make important decisions with regard to what is best for the children they have brought into existence.[7]

This was also the conclusion of the courts in both of the Baby Doe cases and of the physicians in the Johns Hopkins case as well.

Normally, most would agree that the medical treatment of a child is the parents' decision.

Normally, most would agree that the medical treatment of a child is the parents' decision — it is both their right and their obligation. However, the real question is, "Is this an absolute right?" Many would argue that it is a *prima facie* right, and not an absolute right. In other words, in normal situations parents have a right and an obligation concerning decision-making for the medical treatment or nontreatment of their own children. However, that right can be overridden if it comes into conflict with a more fundamental right. In the case of severely impaired newborns, their health and life are more fundamental than the parents' right to choose for them. If the parents' choice severely endangers the health or life of a child, then that right can be overridden. In fact, physicians and the legal system may have a duty to override parents in such cases. Physicians have a duty to "do no harm" to their patients, and the state has a compelling interest in protecting the lives of its citizens.

We recognize such a *prima facie* right in our laws concerning parental care and abuse of children. Richards and Rathbun write in their book *Law and the Physician: A Practical Guide*, "All states have laws that allow children to be treated without the parents' or guardians' consent in special circumstances. These laws are designed to protect either the child or the public health of the community."[8] The kinds of circumstances that they list would be: emergency situations when parents are unavailable, children suspected of being abused or neglected, children with certain communicable diseases, children seeking help for alcohol or drug abuse, and parents who refuse lifesaving medical treatment for their child.

All states have laws that allow children to be treated without the parents' or guardians' consent in special circumstances.

One common reason for the last of these is when parents refuse lifesaving treatment for children due to religious beliefs. For example, Jehovah's Witnesses will not accept blood transfusions. There have been a number of cases when they have refused transfusions for their children. While courts generally honor adult refusal of blood transfusions, they have been disinclined to do the same for children. In *Mitchell v. Davis* (1947) and in *Wallace v. Labrenz* (1952) courts ruled that children should be transfused against the wishes of the parents, reasoning that the parents may have the right to be martyrs themselves, but they cannot force that on their children. This has been the standard ruling in courts concerning parents who refuse treatment to children. Richards and Rathbun explain the normal procedures in such situations:

> The child should be evaluated at once to determine if immediate care is needed. If it is, a judge should be contacted to arrange a temporary guardianship. The child welfare depart-

ment should also be notified because *denying a child necessary medical care is neglect in most states.* . . . Although the court may decide to accede to the parents' religious beliefs, the *physician's duty is to advocate for the child* until the court rules that the child need not be treated.[9]

These situations demonstrate that a parent does not have an absolute right to determine a child's treatment, especially if the parent's decision puts the child's life in danger. Certainly if a parent's right to decide based on religious preferences can be justifiably infringed, then it seems at least plausible that a right to decide based on a desire not to raise a Down's syndrome child, can also be justifiably overridden.

However, many will say, "The situations you raised above are normal healthy children who need emergency care. That is not the case with impaired newborns. There is a *significant difference* between them and the Jehovah's Witnesses cases. This difference is enough to allow parents to decide not to treat severely impaired newborns." What are such "differences"? This brings us to the second moral question: "What basis can be offered to argue that one is justified in forgoing treatment and allowing infants to die?" We will examine three major arguments that have been offered to justify allowing infants to die[10]:

1. *The Nonperson View.* This argument says that the "difference" lies in the status of the infant. Moral rights, especially the right to life, are grounded in being a person, and infants are not persons. They are human beings, but they are not persons in the full sense of the term. One philosopher who holds this view is Michael Tooley. Whether one agrees with Tooley's concept of person or not, he at least is consistent in saying that there is no real difference between an infant and a fetus when it comes to moral rights. However, his point is that neither fetuses nor infants have any moral rights. Tooley holds that there is a condition which an organism must have in order to have a right to life. He writes, "An organism possesses a serious right to life only if it possesses the concept of a self as a continuing subject of experiences and other mental states, and believes that it is itself such a continuing entity."[11]

Tooley calls this the *self-consciousness* requirement. Since infants do not have a self-concept or are not self-conscious they are not persons and therefore there is no moral requirement to treat them.

Tristram Englehardt is another who argues that the infant is not really a person, though for a different reason. Children are not persons in the "strict" sense because they are not adults. Therefore they have no moral rights. He writes:

> Adults belong to themselves in the sense that they are rational and free and therefore responsible for their actions. Adults are *sui juris*. Young children, though, are neither self-possessed nor responsible. While adults exist in and for themselves, as self-directed and self-conscious beings, young children, especially newborn infants, exist for their families and those who love them. They are not, nor can they in any sense be, responsible for themselves. If being a person is to be a responsible agent, a bearer of rights and duties, children are not persons in the strict sense.[12]

There is a difference between functioning as a person and being a person.

How might one respond to these arguments? First, there is a difference between *functioning* as a person and *being* a person. We referred to this argument in Chapter 2 when some attempted to deny the personhood of the fetus. A functionalistic definition of personhood fails because there are many times people do not function *as* persons, and yet we would still consider them to *be* persons. A person does not have a self-concept nor is self-conscious when she is sleeping or under an anaesthetic. Neither is she "self-possessed" or "responsible." For example, if a person sleepwalks and breaks an item while sleepwalking, we do not hold him "responsible" for his actions, but this hardly means they were not a person at the time, though one could argue they may not have been functioning as one. It is possible to be a person and not function as one.

Second, the basic inherent capacity for functioning as a person is present from conception. In other words, the essence of personhood is present from conception, through birth, and throughout all of a human being's life. An infant has this basic capacity in a latent undeveloped form. If proper care is given to him, he will grow and develop as a person. In severely impaired infants this development might be suppressed due to neurological damage. However, that does not mean it is not there. The only time a human organism ceases to have personhood is when it has died. Personhood is there by nature of what kind of being it is.

Third, this view goes counter to some of our most basic intuitions. For example, Tooley suggests that it is possible for a normal adult animal to have more worth than a defective infant because some higher-level animals can have more of a self-concept than an infant. However, most people recognize that there is something inherent about man that makes him different from other animals. Christians would argue that it is because we are image-of-God bearers. Therefore morality applies to us in a way different from other animals.[13] This also goes counter to the way we intuitively treat infants: as persons having value. Englehardt gives the impression that an infant's only value is in being "possessed" by a family. However, persons aren't possessions. They have intrinsic value of their own.

Finally, if infants are not persons, then why kill only severely impaired newborns? Why not kill or experiment on any newborn before it has developed into a person? If they are not persons then, in fact, none of them have any moral rights. Both Tooley and Englehardt apply their arguments only to severely impaired newborns. However, if they were consistent, it would not be morally wrong for any parent to kill or allow *any* child to die for *any* reason including economic reasons or sex selection.

2. *Quality-of-Life Arguments*. Some have argued that the "difference" between healthy and impaired children lies in the

quality of life that an infant might have to face if he is allowed to live. The basic argument is that it is morally justifiable to withdraw or withhold treatment from a severely impaired infant if its present or future quality of life will drop below a certain threshold. Those who hold this view argue that life is a relative good, not an absolute good. It is good relative only to the quality of life it achieves. It is possible that one's quality of life could be worse than death itself. At that point withholding/withdrawing treatment could be justifiable. Quality of life can be based on a number of different criteria, however two criteria will be noted.

> *"Quality of life" proponents argue that life is a relative good, not an absolute good.*

Richard McCormick has argued that the standard should be "relational potential," or the ability to have meaningful relationships. For McCormick the question is, "Granted we can easily save the life, but what kind of a life are we saving?"[14] McCormick's view is that:

> Life is not a value to be preserved in and for itself. To maintain that would commit us to a form of medical vitalism that makes no human or Judeo-Christian sense. It is a value to be preserved precisely as a condition for other values, and therefore insofar as these other values remain attainable. Since these other values cluster around and are rooted in human relationships, it seems to follow that life is a value to be preserved only insofar as it contains some potentiality for human relationships.[15]

Therefore, McCormick would hold that any infant who lacks the potential for future relationships can be said to have no interests and therefore has a low enough quality of life that one can justifiably allow it to die.

Another criterion for quality of life can be found in a research project on care of imperiled newborns sponsored by the Hastings Center. Participants argued that withholding or withdrawing life-sustaining treatment from impaired infants should be determined primarily using a **"best interest standard"** for the infant. The best interest standard would be applied under three possible conditions: the infant is dying, treatment is medically contraindicated, or continued life would be worse than death. Concerning this last condition they state, "The third condition opens the door to quality of life considerations, but requires that such conditions be viewed *from the infant's point of view*. That is, certain states of being, marked by severe and intractable pain and suffering, can be viewed as worse than death."[16] Therefore, in considerations of "best interests" for the severely impaired infant, he or she can be allowed to die.

The criteria in determining "quality of life" are too vague and subjective.

One can make a number of responses to the quality of life argument. First, the criteria in determining "quality of life" are too vague and subjective, rendering this determination difficult to use as a moral basis for allowing an infant to die. John A. Robertson comments, "Comparisons of relative worth among persons, or between persons and other interests, raise moral and methodological issues that make any argument that relies on such comparisons extremely vulnerable."[17] There are several reasons why it is difficult to make these kinds of judgments. First, different people mean different things by a "low quality of life," and there is just no way a proxy can know what the "infant's view" would be. Second, the people who are making this judgment on the infant, usually the parents and physician, are themselves dealing with the impact of treatment on their *own* interests, and therefore it's unrealistic to expect them to make a disinterested objective assessment of what the infant's interests might be. Third, our view of quality of life changes throughout our life. Some restrictions we wouldn't accept at one time might not be so unacceptable at another time. Oftentimes a particular state of affairs we think we could never live with, turns out not to be as bad as we had thought. Fourth, we make quality-of-life judgments based on our own personal experiences of a life already lived. But an impaired infant may never share such experiences and so that judgment might be completely different for her because she has no basis for comparison. For a person who has spent life with sight, blindness would be a terrible loss that may impact him deeply. People who have been blind all their lives don't experience the loss in the same way. The same could be said of the loss of ambulatory abilities or of being mentally retarded. This doesn't mean such disabilities aren't tragic in an objective sense, but it is to say that they are not experienced the same way by all and therefore a proxy quality-of-life judgment is very difficult to assess. In light of these considerations, we need to acknowledge that there is just too much subjectivity to weigh proxy quality-of-life judgments heavily.

> *It is logically impossible to demonstrate that death is better than life.*

A second problem with the quality-of-life argument is that it is logically impossible to demonstrate that death is better than life. We need to note what is being claimed here. Those offering this argument are not saying that eternal life or the after-life is better than present life, they are saying that *nonexistence* is better than *existence*. Now what precisely is "nonexistence"? It is simply nothing. That is why there is a logical problem. The problem is that when you compare two things, you are comparing their properties or characteristics. When you make a valuative claim, that thing "A" is better than thing

"B," you are saying that the characteristics of one are in some way superior to the characteristics of the other. However, "nothing" does not have any characteristics. Therefore, there is no basis for comparison between something and nothing; you can't compare something to nothing because there is "nothing" to compare it to. One can logically never make the claim that something is better than nothing or that nothing is better than something. Therefore to claim that a particular state of life, a "painful" state, is "worse than death" simply does not follow. It is incoherent.

Third, the quality-of-life argument involves a view of persons that is seriously flawed. Christian philosopher J.P. Moreland writes that this view "fails to treat persons as entities with intrinsic value simply as human beings, and it tends to reduce the value of human beings to their social utility or to a view of humans as bundles of pleasant mental and physical states or capacities."[18] The impression is given that the only times persons have value are when they can have certain states like "relationships" or "freedom from pain." If one loses one of these states, then his value as a person is in jeopardy. However, persons have inherent and intrinsic value by nature of what they are. We do not say the mentally retarded are less valuable than the highly intelligent just because the mentally retarded cannot experience relationships at the same level as the intelligent. To say so would be elitist thinking and the height of arrogance. One is reminded of the Ghost of Christmas Present chiding Scrooge, "It may be in the sight of Heaven, you are more worthless and less fit to live than millions like this poor man's child."

Fourth, "the presence of suffering is simply not enough, by itself, to signal the presence of a morally inappropriate situation."[19] No one denies that all should be done to relieve as much suffering as possible, both presently and in the future. But as we have said in previous chapters, relief of suffering is not a mandate justifying one to do *any* action in the name of relief of suffering. Suffering itself, while it is an evil, is not always morally bad. It is not enough to warrant the overriding of our accepted norms concerning treatment of the nondying.

Fifth, quality-of-life judgments can simply be wrong. Robertson comments that "the margin of error in such predications may be very great."[20] Even McCormick admits this; in fact his admission and response is somewhat surprising:

> Because this guideline [relational capacity] is precisely that, mistakes will be made. Some infants will be judged in all sincerity to be devoid of any meaningful relational potential when that is actually not quite the case. This risk of error should not lead to abandonment of decisions; for that is to walk away from the human scene. Risk of error means only that we must proceed with great humility, caution, and tentativeness. Concretely, it means that if err we must at times, it is better to err on the side of life — and therefore tilt in that direction.[21]

What McCormick is saying about erring on the "side of life" is not that we should, in the face of doubt, allow severely impaired newborns to live, but that we should allow them to die because they cannot *really* live any kind of qualitative life. We can see examples of the mistakes that have been made. The parents of Kerri-Lynn were told that she would be paralyzed, retarded and vulnerable to infections for the rest of her life which would probably not go much beyond a few painful years, if that long. Yet she is not anywhere near the condition that was predicted. Dax Cowart, the fire-burned victim I mentioned in a previous chapter, wanted to end his life because he thought it would be completely meaningless. He had lost his sight, the use of his hands and was badly disfigured. Today he is a successful lawyer, married, and generally happy. Many Down's syndrome children live happy and meaningful lives for many years. Therefore, one needs to approach quality-of-life predictions with extreme caution.

One needs to approach quality-of-life predictions with extreme caution.

Finally, the principle of justice demands that we protect the weakest in society. What a severely impaired child needs are those who are caring and looking out for her or his needs. There is a subtle form of discrimination under the guise of care in not treating impaired infants. As we saw in the Johns Hopkins and Baby Doe cases, if the child had been normal, the medical procedures they needed would have been performed without a second thought. However, because of their impaired condition the parents were allowed to deny that care. That is discriminatory treatment and goes against our practice of equal protection under the law.

   3. *The Harms-to-Others Argument.* Finally some argue that the "difference" between healthy and severely impaired infants must take into account not only the suffering of the infant, but the suffering of others who are impacted by this tragic circumstance. The most obvious group of people are the parents and immediate family members. They will have to raise the child and care for it in its impaired condition. This will place a great emotional, psychological, and financial burden on the family. Tristram Englehardt, Jr. notes the importance of "costs" to the family:

> The accent is on the absence of a positive duty to treat in the presence of severe inconvenience (costs) to the parents; treatment that is very costly is not obligatory. What is suggested here is a general notion that there is never a duty to engage in extraordinary treatment and that "extraordinary" can be defined in terms of costs. This argument concerns children (1) whose future quality of life is likely to be seriously compromised and (2) whose present treatment would be very costly. The issue is that of the circumstances under which parents would not be obliged to take on severe burdens on behalf of their children or those circumstances under which society would not be so obligated.[22]

Carson Strong argues even more firmly that "when a heavy burden would fall on the family with the survival of an impaired newborn, it is permissible to put the interests of the family above those of the infant."[23]

   Not only will the family suffer, but others will suffer as well. Society will need to spend more resources on this child than the average person, therefore the impaired infant is receiving more than his or her fair share, leaving less for others. Also in some way the physicians and nurses suffer though not to the same degree as the family. There is a lot of strain in the NICU taking care of impaired newborns. Physicians may feel their skills are being misused in caring for an impaired newborn. Therefore due to these harms to others, the nontreatment of the severely impaired newborn is justified.

The costs to the parents and family or society are weighed as greater than the life of the child.

The first problem with considering these kinds of harms is that this is based on a utilitarian type of calculation. In weighing the benefits and burdens, the costs to the parents and family or society are weighed as greater than the life of the child and therefore the child's life is sacrificed for the good of the family or society. However, as you might remember from our discussion in the first chapter, utilitarian calculations are very problematical. First, there is the incommensurability problem. The judgment that the benefits of family outweigh the infant's interests "requires a coherent way of measuring and comparing interpersonal utilities."[24] Yet there does not seem to be any way to accomplish this. Second, a common problem with utilitarian calculations is that people get treated as means to ends rather than ends themselves. The value of the infant is now placed in terms of costs or benefits for the family or society. The infant is not being treated as a person itself, intrinsically valuable. Robertson writes, "If the life of one individual, however useless, may be sacrificed for the benefit of any person, however useful, or for the benefit of any number of persons, then we have acknowledged the principle that rational utility may justify any outcome . . . we reach the point where protection of life depends solely on social judgments of utility."[25]

Second, what criteria for judging between the family's/ society's needs and the baby's life are offered? Not only is such comparison not possible due to incommensurability, but the criteria to use in making the comparison are highly debatable. How much burden on the family justifies not treating the infant? Financial costs of continued care? The cost of a mother having to give up a career to care for an impaired child? Major adjustments in home life? The problem is that a whole range of burdens are possible, and it would be very difficult to regulate which ones are enough to allow the infant to die and which are not. Because there are no clear objective criteria for balancing the burdens of treating the infant with the benefits of not treating the infant, treatment cannot be justifiably withheld from newborns. One needs to have justifiable reasons to take an innocent life, but none are offered here.

One needs to have justifiable reasons to take an innocent life, but none are offered here.

Third, parents have a filial obligation to care for their children and the fact that the children are impaired does not negate that obligation; in fact that obligation is stronger because the need is greater. If the "harms to others" argument really worked the way proponents suggest, then why stop with impaired newborns? Why not argue that parents may do away with their children any time they become too much of a burden? Why does he have to be suffering? It is not the child's suffering that is the thrust of this argument, it is that he or she is a burden. Therefore, any time the child is a burden I should be allowed to dispose of it. Most recognize the lunacy of such a suggestion. Part of the basis of family morality is that parents have obligations to children which they cannot neglect purely because the child is now a burden. As we said in our abortion chapter, child abuse, neglect and abandonment laws recognize this obligation. That is why Congress placed medical neglect under the Child Abuse Prevention and Treatment Act of 1973. It states, "The term 'medical neglect' includes, but is not limited to, the withholding of medically indicated treatment from a disabled infant with a life-threatening condition."[26]

None of this is to deny the devastating impact an impaired child can have on a family. The initial effect always carries feelings of guilt, grief, and loss of dignity to the parents. Adjustments must be made in the home which cause anxiety and tension among all family members. There is a significant drain on financial resources as they care for the infant. However, it is not a hopeless situation. Counseling is available to deal with the adjustments and initial feeling. Resources are often available to help in caring for the infant. For Christians such an experience can be positive as one learns how to live sacrificially for another. This is not to downplay the real difficulty of such a situation, but, "Suffering there is, but seldom is it so overwhelming or so imminent that the only alternative is death of the child."[27]

Passive Euthanasia and the Impaired Newborn

Is there ever a time when nontreatment is justified for an impaired infant? The answer is yes — when the infant is dying. If the infant is not dying, then medical treatment should be given. Such a view has been called a "medical indications" or "medical feasibility" view. It has been held by a number of people, but perhaps the most well known proponent was the Christian ethicist Paul Ramsey. Richard Sparks summarizes Ramsey's position well:

> If a patient, competent or otherwise, has entered the dying process, in which all curative efforts are futile or at best serve only minimally to forestall the *imminently* inevitable, then such medical procedures are optional, perhaps even contraindicated. . . In the cases of patients, competent or incompetent, who are not irreversibly dying, a medical indications policy asserts that any treatment that prognastically will be medically beneficial is automatically morally indicated.[28]

It is important to remember the distinction between passive and active euthanasia.

It is important for a moment to return to our discussion in a previous chapter (Chapter 3) of the distinction between passive and active euthanasia. In that chapter we made the distinction that active euthanasia involves both (1) the intention of death and (2) that the direct actions of the agent are the cause of death of the patient. Passive euthanasia occurs when (1) the intention is not the death of the patient, but relief of the burdens of treatment and (2) it is not the direct action of the agent that is the cause of death, but the particular debilitation. This distinction is somewhat blurred in the case of nontreatment of the impaired newborn. In this case, it is the withholding or withdrawing of treatment of the newborn that is the direct cause of death. While this might be interpreted as passive, in this case it is active because in normal cases such treatment would be beneficial without being excessively burdensome. Ramsey makes this point:

> When care is not even attempted in the case of defective nondying infants, there is no morally significant distinction, between action and abstention. Morally what in this case is not done is the same as doing. The benign neglect of defective infants — who are not dying, who cannot themselves refuse treatment, who are most in need of human help — is the same as directly dispatching them: involuntary euthanasia.[29]

Examples of the kinds of cases that might normally fit into the "dying" category would be extremely premature infants of which even strongly aggressive therapy would be futile, and possibly anencephalic infants (which will be discussed more below). In these cases palliative and comfort care should be maintained, but aggressive life-saving care would not be warranted. Examples of the kinds of cases that would generally not be considered dying would be children born with Down's syndrome, mentally retarded children, spina bifida children, or children born with physical, but not life-threatening, deformities. All judgments concerning the dying/nondying status of the impaired infant are medical judgments and it needs to be readily admitted that such cases are not always clear. However, once a judgment is medically determined, the infant's status of dying/nondying becomes the determining factor concerning treatment, not quality of life, third party considerations, or personhood.

There are a number of reasons to support this view. First, it preserves the basic moral notion that all human persons have intrinsic worth and grounds that worth in being a member of a natural kind, humankind. It holds to the mandate not to kill innocent persons without just cause. The fact that the infant is deformed or impaired is not a justifiable cause for its death. Second, it avoids the vagueness and subjectivity of both the quality-of-life view and the nonperson view. We are no longer trying to decipher what the "best interests are from the infant's point of view." We are also rejecting the functionalistic concept of personhood for an essential concept of personhood. Third, it places the focus on the person and on the treatment instead of discriminating between the morally irrelevant properties of severely impaired infants and healthy infants. Ramsey comments:

> This requires no comparison of patient-*persons* or of different stages or conditions of the same patient-person in order to determine his quality-of-life struggles or prospects. It requires simply a *comparison of treatments* to determine whether any are likely to be beneficial in any way other than prolonging dying.[30]

Finally, this view places the discussion of nontreatment within the broader area of euthanasia instead of specifically pinpointing infants. One can treat infants like adults in evaluating their treatment. We allow adults to die when we recognize that care is no longer of benefit and there is nothing more that can be done. There is no reason not to treat infants the same way.

Anencephalics — A Special Case?

In recent years several physicians and ethicists have attempted to argue that the anencephalic child is such a special case that it needs to be considered apart from the other forms of impairment we have discussed thus far. Merely the fact that this has been raised calls for a separate discussion.

What is anencephaly? The word literally means "no brain," however that might communicate the wrong idea. Anencephaly results from a failure of the neural tissue to completely close at the *cephalic* or top end of the neural system. This closure normally occurs between the second and third week of pregnancy. The cerebral cortex or upper level of the brain is missing but the brain stem is always present. Infants born with anencephaly usually do not have a closed cranium and one can often look into the head and see the missing cephalus and exposed brain stem. The brain stem is that part of the brain which controls the involuntary operations of heart rate, lungs, blood pressure, salt and water balance, kidneys and other organs and systems. However, the cerebral cortex contains the area where such operations as consciousness, memories, purposive action, emotional states, social abilities and, some believe, sentience take place. Therefore, while the infant is definitely alive, it has no capacity, nor ever will have a capacity, for functioning as a person.

> *The question concerning anencephalics has to do with their status as persons.*

Anencephaly occurs in about 1,000 pregnancies per year and is usually diagnosed during pregnancy. About 95% of these are aborted even though there is a possibility of misdiagnosis. Of those carried to term, about half are stillborn.[31] Those anencephalics who survive through birth rarely live for more than a week, often dying because of the exposure of the brain stem. However, some have been known to live longer due to special care. In fact one source writes, "If the brain were sufficiently protected, life could be prolonged for years."[32] The question concerning anencephalics has to do with their status as persons and the medical status of their treatment.

These questions arise because of a number of cases concerning anencephalics that have occurred in recent years, especially two that have been through the legal system.

1. *In the Matter of Theresa Ann Campo Pearson.* On March 21, 1992, Theresa Ann Campo Pearson was born to Laura Campo and Justin Pearson, an unmarried couple, in Fort Lauderdale, Florida. Because Laura did not have medical insurance, she did not find out until the eighth month of pregnancy that her baby was anencephalic, which was deemed too late for an abortion. Laura claims that had she known earlier she would have aborted the child. However, Laura had heard about the possibility of organ donation from anencephalics and decided to carry the baby to term and then have its organs donated so that some good could come from this tragic situation.

The idea of organ donation from anencephalics has been a topic of debate within the medical community for some time.

The idea of organ donation from anencephalics has been a topic of debate within the medical community for some time. There is a desperate need for organs for infants, and such organs need to come from other infants. The problem is that in the normal course of dying, the blood flow slows down as the heart gradually begins to stop beating. Organs suffer from a lack of oxygen and begin to rapidly deteriorate becoming unusable for transplantation. However, if the organs were excised from a breathing infant, then they would stand a much better chance in a successful transplantation. After birth anencephalics could be placed on a ventilator to insure that the organs remained oxygenated. A determination could be made that the infant was brain dead and then organs could be excised and transplanted into other infants. At least one transplantation from an anencephalic had taken place previously at Loma Linda Hospital in California. This was what Laura and Justin wanted for Theresa.

The problem was that Theresa was not brain dead. Upon birth Theresa was placed on a ventilator. After one week the ventilator was removed and she could breathe on her own for a period of time, indicating that the brain stem was still functioning. Laura and Justin requested to have Theresa declared legally dead so that her organs could be removed for transplantation. However, the hospital refused, claiming that, according to Florida State Law which uses the Harvard Criteria for whole brain death, Theresa was not officially brain dead and organs cannot be excised from a living human being. Laura and Justin then petitioned the circuit court of Broward County for a declaratory judgment stating that Theresa was legally dead. The circuit court denied their request citing, again, that Theresa was not brain dead according to state law. The case was heard on appeal and the appellate court affirmed the lower court's ruling. However, the case was referred to the Florida State Supreme Court due to its significance.

Theresa died on March 30, 1992, before the case came before the State Supreme Court. However, the court agreed to review the case and, on November 12, 1992, rendered a unanimous opinion on the question: "Is an anencephalic newborn considered 'dead' for purposes of organ donation solely by reason of its congenital deformity?" The court held that "as a matter of Florida common law the cardiopulmonary definition of death should be applied in cases involving anencephaly that survive without life support." Under this definition of death, Theresa was alive as long as her lungs and heart spontaneously functioned and therefore she could not be used for organ transplantation.

2. *In the Matter of Baby K.* On October 13, 1992, Stephanie Keene, an anencephalic infant, was born in Fairfax Hospital in Falls Church, Virginia. As is normal with anencephalics, she was placed on a respirator. Stephanie had been prenatally diagnosed with anencephaly, but her mother, being a Christian, refused to have an abortion. As was the case with Theresa, the mother and father were unmarried and were referred to throughout the case as Ms. H and Mr. K. Stephanie's father remained only distantly involved in the case.

Within days of Stephanie's birth, hospital medical personnel approached Ms. H and requested that a "Do Not Resuscitate (**DNR**) Order" be placed in Stephanie's file allowing for disconnection of the ventilator and the subsequent death of Stephanie. DNR's are standard procedures in hospitals when it is determined that resuscitative efforts would be futile and only prolong the dying process. The medical personnel explained that no treatment existed for her daughter's condition, that she would never be able to function as a person, and that the ventilator was therefore medically unnecessary and inappropriate. However, Ms. H declined to agree to the DNR order stating her belief that God could work a miracle. The hospital then asked the hospital ethics committee to assist in overriding the mother's wishes. The committee met with Ms. H on Oct. 22, 1992 and again attempted to convince her that such care was futile and to allow the hospital to disconnect the ventilator. Ms. H refused to follow the ethics committee's recommendation.

The hospital attempted to circumvent legal action by transferring Stephanie to a nursing home during a period when she was not in need of ventilator support. Ms. H agreed to move Stephanie only on the condition that should she develop respiratory distress, the hospital would take her back. Stephanie was transferred to the nursing home on Nov. 30 during a period when the ventilator was not necessary. However over the next several months Stephanie needed to be returned to the hospital twice due to respiratory distress. After the second of these visits, when Stephanie was returned to the nursing home on April 13, the hospital decided to seek a court order allowing them to discontinue treatment to Stephanie. The case went before federal Judge Claude Hilton and became known as the "Baby K" case.

On July 1, 1993, Judge Hilton ruled that the hospital had a duty to provide full medical care to Stephanie. He appealed to the Americans with Disabilities Act of 1990, The Rehabilitation Act of 1973, and the Emergency Medical Treatment and Active Labor Act (EMTALA) in his decision. The case was appealed and in December 1994 the Fourth Circuit

Court of Appeals upheld Judge Hilton's ruling specifically stating that the EMTALA did not make an exception for anencephalics. The case was appealed to the United States Supreme Court which let stand the Fourth Circuit's ruling.

> ## EMTALA did not make an exception for anencephalics.

During the Fourth Circuit trial, Laura Flint from Jacksonville, Florida, appeared on behalf of Ms. H. She had given birth to an anencephalic daughter who lived beyond the age of four years old before dying. Mrs. Flint reported that her daughter was able to recognize voices, see colors, hold up her head and push toys. She showed pictures of her daughter sitting on Santa's lap and in front of a birthday cake. She stated "To me it was worth it every day we had with her."[33] Stephanie herself lived until she was two and a half. She died in April 1995, and her mother contended throughout her life that life was precious and that only God could take her daughter.

Cases like those above have raised serious moral questions about the status of anencephalics. Since such children are born without even the capacity to function as persons, should they be considered persons or not? Should the standard for brain death be changed to include neocortical death? If anenecephalics are considered persons, what kind of medical treatment should they receive?

Concerning the first of these questions, there are those who suggest that the anencephalic infant is not a person. Gregory Pence doesn't even argue the issue, but simply states, "Nevertheless, anencephaly is the most serious of all birth defects, because the baby essentially lacks the higher brain necessary for personhood."[34] While he does not comment on anencephalics specifically, Christian theologian Robert Rakestraw might take this view as it follows from his view on PVS patients. He holds that, "Neocortical destruction is both a necessary and sufficient condition for declaring an individual dead theologically."[35] Certainly if personal life ends with the destruction of the neocortex, it must not be there if the neocortex is never present. One group of physicians summarizes this position well:

> Valuable human life is intrinsically related to higher brain function, or at least the potential of developing it. Brainstem function and artificial life support could maintain the bodies of anencephalic infants, but would not give them what most people consider to be meaningful life as human beings. Hence, it is morally right to differentiate between biologic human life and personal life. Anencephalic infants may be living human beings, but they lack personhood.[36]

While it is possible that personhood is never in fact present in the anencephalic, we should approach the status of the anencephalic with extreme caution. There are several reasons for holding this view. First, the anencephalic is still a living, breathing human being. Human beings by nature are persons due to the kind of beings they are. Unless there is overwhelming evidence, that nature should be presumed to be present.

Human beings by nature are persons due to the kind of beings they are.

Second, one should be careful about identifying personhood so strongly with any specific part of brain. While it seems that the absence of the neocortex means that certain capacities for functioning as a person may not be present, it does not rule out the possibility that the basic inherent capacity may be rooted more deeply in the entire neural system. The fact that an anencephalic may not be able to realize these capacities does not mean they are not present. Stephen Schwartz refers to these as "latent capacities" and his comment is worth repeating here:

Even a very severely abnormal or handicapped human being has the basic inherent capacity to function as a person, which is a sign that he is a person. The abnormality represents a *hindrance* to the actual working of this capacity, to its manifestation in actual functioning. It does not imply the *absence* of this capacity, as in a non-person.[37]

Third, those who hold that anenecephalics should be declared nonpersons in order to excise organs for donation often make a point that anenecephalics do not feel pain. However, this is a highly questionable premise. Dr. Alan Shewmon, considered the world's greatest authority on anencephalics, states:

It simply begs the question to state categorically that [anencephalic babies] lack conscious awareness because they lack cerebral hemispheres. Much less is there any logical or physiological basis for the claim of some that an anencephalic infant can neither feel, nor experience, pain "by definition." For practical purposes, one should presume, at the very least, that anencephalic babies are no less aware or capable of suffering than some laboratory animals with even smaller brains, which everyone seems to feel obliged to treat "humanely."[38]

In short, it is possible that anenecephalics do feel pain, and if so, they should be granted at least minimum humane treatment.

Stephanie Keene lived two and a half years and the child of Laura Flint lived until four and exhibited some possible traits of personhood.

Fourth, while rare, there have been cases of anenecephalics who have lived longer than the few days usually predicted. Stephanie Keene lived two and a half years and the child of Laura Flint lived until four and exhibited some possible traits of personhood. There are other cases where anencephalics have lived for a year or longer. When one considers these cases in light of the above comment that if the brain were protected they could go on for years, it should give one pause in automatically jumping to the conclusion that such infants are not persons or should be harvested for organs. Some have claimed that such cases are simply misdiagnoses, and true anencephalics by definition will not live that long. However, if that is true, it only makes the case stronger for not using such infants for donations — in case there is a misdiagnosis.

Fifth, if one changes the criterion for death from whole brain death to neocortical death, which would include anenecephalics, many believe there is a danger of slipping down the slope to including many other areas where absence of a functioning person might lead to termination of life. Some say that anenecephalics are sufficiently similar to other debilitations, such as PVS, hydrocephaly, atelencephaly, degenerative brain disorders, profound retardation and advanced Alzheimer's, that a clear distinction may not be seen, such that these may also be grouped in with those considered neocortically dead. If personhood is lacking in the anencephalic, perhaps it is lacking in these disorders also. If one argues that we would only change the definition to include anencaphalics, then one also has to ask if it is worth creating a whole separate category and changing a basic definition for such a small number of beings. It is estimated that only about 300 anencephalics per year can be potential organ donors.[39] The increase in supply of organs for transplantation would be minimal.

Many believe there is a danger of slipping down a very slippery slope.

Enough evidence exists that warrants that the benefit of the doubt should be given to the anencephalic child concerning personhood. While it is possible that personhood is absent, enough evidence is not available to suggest this. The benefit of the doubt should always go toward maintaining life if there is ever a reasonable question.

However, now there is the question as to the anencephalic child's medical status. This is a question in which a medical judgment is necessary and such a judgment lies outside the scope of this book. In general, however, Gilbert Meilaender's assessment for the normal care for anencephalics is acceptable:

> How would we ordinarily care for this baby at her birth? The case suggests a standard, and it seems to me the right one: she would receive "no aggressive treatment in the neonatal nursery." She is born dying, and proper care for her does not entail useless attempts to sustain her life.[40]

Usually this would mean that once born the anencephalic would be placed on a respirator. After a period of time in the medical judgment of physicians, it would be determined if he or she were brain dead. As long as the infant remained alive, ordinary care should be used to maintain her or his life. However, aggressive care should be avoided. Again there comes a time to recognize that there is nothing more that we can do.

Conclusion   We need to revisit a recurring theme in the two previous chapters of this book. It is the theme of "caring, but not killing." It is the recognition that God has placed limits on how much we can do. Those limits inform us when we can do no more and when medical care must end. However, the same limits also inform us that we cannot kill infants through non-treatment and justifying it as a way of healing. Certainly many of those who desire to end the lives of their children are acting out of pure motives. Wanting to end suffering, avoid a life of misery, or, in the case of anencephalics, to cause some good to come from a tragic situation is understandable. Nevertheless some are acting from less honorable motives, such as not wanting to be hassled with the raising of an impaired child, though surely most persons are not feeling this way. But as good as those motives are, we cannot ever intend the death of another person. That is a role meant only for the Lord of life, and we must not usurp it.

No one can even pretend to be able to answer the question of why God allows some children to come into the world with the disabilities we have discussed in this chapter. But God does give us guidance for how we are to treat them. We see it modeled in the parable of the good Samaritan. There we observe a person who was severely beaten and in dire need of help. The Samaritan, whom our Lord praises, went out of his way to care. He was the good neighbor to this man. Surely if he can be such a neighbor to a perfect stranger, we can be so to our own children. The Christian ethicist Paul Ramsey said,

> Persons are not to be reducible for their potential. Patients are to be loved and cared for no matter who they are and no matter what their potential for higher values is, and certainly not on account of their responsiveness. Who they are, in Christian ethical perspective, is our neighbors. They do not become nearer neighbors because of any capacity they own, nor lesser neighbors because they lack some ability to prevail in their struggle for human achievement.[41]

ENDNOTES

[1]Quoted in Gregory Pence, *Classic Cases in Medical Ethics*, 2nd ed. (New York: McGraw-Hill, 1995), p.181.

[2]National Center for Health Statistics, 1995 and 1996 averages.

[3]NCHS, 1995 statistics.

[4]Pence, *Classic Cases*, pp. 175-177.

[5]Pence, *Classic Cases*, p. 178.

[6]Kathleen Kerr, "Proving Their Prognosis Wrong, Baby Jane Doe Busy Learning, Laughing," *Newsday* (September 20, 1990), p. 7.

[7]Patricia Phillips, "Parents Alone Have the Right to Decide If Infant Euthanasia Is Ethical," in *Euthanasia: Opposing Viewpoints*, ed. by Carol Wekesser (San Diego: Greenhaven Press, 1995), p. 187.

[8]Edward P. Richards III, JD, and Katharine C. Rathbun, MD, *Law and the Physician: A Practical Guide* (Boston: Little, Brown & Co, 1993), p. 170.

[9]Richards and Rathbun, *Law*, p. 166.

[10]I am grateful to my colleague and friend, Dr. J.P. Moreland, for his appraisal of these arguments. Much of the material I am presenting here is based on his analysis of these positions as found in his chapter "Infanticide" in *The Life and Death Debate: Moral Issues of Our Time*, with Norman L. Geisler (Westport, CT: Greenwood Press, 1990).

[11]Michael Tooley, "Abortion and Infanticide"(1972) reprinted in *Classic Works in Medical Ethics*, ed. by Gregory Pence (New York: McGraw-Hill, 1998), p. 206.

[12]Tristram Englehardt, "Aiding the Death of Young Children: Ethical Issues" (1975), reprinted in *Last Rights: Assisted Suicide and Euthanasia Debated*, ed. by Michael Uhlmann (Grand Rapids: Eerdmans, 1998), p. 390.

[13]I am not arguing that we have no moral obligations to animals. I believe that we do have certain obligations. For example, we cannot cruelly torture animals. Our obligation to our environment is the recognition that God has given it to us and we are to be proper caretakers of it and respect it as his creation. While Scripture allows the slaying of animals for food and clothing, they are never to be needlessly tortured.

[14]Richard McCormick, "To Save or Let Die: The Dilemma of Modern Medicine"(1974), reprinted in *Biomedical Ethics*, 2nd ed., ed. by Thomas A. Mappes and Jane S. Zembaty (New York: McGraw-Hill, 1986), p. 431.

[15]Ibid., p. 431.

[16]Members of The Hastings Center Research Project on the Care of Impaired Newborns, "Standards of Judgment for Treatment of Imperiled Newborns"(1987), reprinted in *Biomedical Ethics*, 4th ed., ed. by Thomas A. Mappes and David Degrazia (New York: McGraw-Hill, 1996), p. 423, emphasis added.

[17]John A. Robertson, "Involuntary Euthanasia of Defective Newborns" (1975), reprinted in *Classic Works in Medical Ethics: Core Philosophical Readings*, ed. by Gregory Pence (New York: McGraw-Hill, 1998), p. 223.

[18]Moreland, "Infanticide," p. 52.

[19]Ibid.

[20]Robertson, "Involuntary Euthanasia," p. 224.

[21]McCormick, "To Save," p. 432.

[22]Englehardt, "Aiding the Death," p. 392.

[23]Carson Strong, "The Neonatologist's Duty to Patient and Parents," *Hastings Center Report* 14 (August 1984), p. 13.

[24]Robertson, "Involuntary Euthanasia," p. 225.

[25]Ibid.

[26]Final Rule: 45 CFR 1340. U.S. Department of Health and Human Services (1985).

[27]Robertson, "Involuntary Euthanasia," p. 227.

[28]Richard C. Sparks, C.S.P., *To Treat or Not to Treat: Bioethics and the Handicapped Newborn* (Mahwah, NJ: Paulist Press, 1988), pp. 34, 37, emphasis his.

[29]Paul Ramsey, *Ethics at the Edges of Life: Medical and Legal Intersections* (New Haven, CT: Yale University Press, 1978), p. 195.

[30]Ibid., p. 178.

[31]Statistics from Pence, *Classic Cases*, p. 327.

[32]Paul A. Byrne, M.D., Joseph C. Evers, M.D., and Richard G. Nilges, M.D., "Anencephaly — Organ Donation?" *Issues in Law and Medicine*, 9:1 (Summer 1993), p. 32.

[33]The story of Laura Flint's appearance is from "Baby K's right to life rests in court's hands," by Lori Sharn, *USA Today* (Oct 27, 1993), p. 11A.

[34]Pence, *Classic Cases*, p. 327.

[35]Robert. V. Rakestraw "The Persistent Vegetative State and the Withdrawal of Nutrition and Hydration" (1992), reprinted in *Readings in Christian Ethics*, ed. by David K. Clark and Robert V. Rakestraw (Grand Rapids: Baker, 1996), p. 128. In a personal correspondence with Dr. Rakestraw, he stated that he was "not willing to say that they [anencephalics] are not persons because their condition is not able to be diagnosed and monitored as precisely as PVS patients." He stated that he would not support an abortion of an anencephalic because the diagnosis is not without error. He goes on to say that "If the newborn was really like a PVS patient and this could be determined with certainty, then I see no need for artificial sustenance" (February 9, 1999).

[36]Avraham Steinberg, MD, Eliezer Katz, MD, and Charles L. Sprung, MD, "Use of anenecephalics as organ donors," *Critical Care Medicine* (November 1993), p. 1788. It is unclear whether this is the position of the authors themselves.

[37]Stephen Schwartz, *The Moral Question of Abortion* (Chicago: Loyola University Press, 1990), p. 97 (emphasis mine).

[38]Quoted in Byrne, et al., pp. 32-33.

[39]Steinberg, et al., p. 1788.

[40]Gilbert Meilaender, "The Anencephalic Newborn as Organ Donor — Commentary," *Hastings Center Report*, 16:2 (April 1986), p. 23.

[41]Ramsey, *Ethics*, p. 185.

References

Works on Imperiled Newborns. (Many of the references from the two previous chapters have information that would apply here as well.)

Lammers, Stephen E. and Allen Verhey, eds. *On Moral Medicine: Theological Perspectives in Medical Ethics*. Grand Rapids: Eerdmans, 1987. Chapter 15.

Mappes, Thomas A. and David Degrazia, eds. *Biomedical Ethics*. 4th ed. New York: McGraw-Hill, 1996. Chapter 7.

McMillan, Richard C., H. Tristram Engelhardt, Jr., and Stuart F. Spicker, eds. *Euthanasia and the Newborn: Conflicts Regarding Saving Lives*. Boston: D. Reidel Publishers, 1987.

Moreland, J.P. and Norman L. Geisler. *The Life and Death Debate: Moral Issues of Our Time*. Westport, CT: Greenwood Press, 1990. Chapter 3.

Munson, Ronald. *Intervention and Reflection: Basic Issues in Medical Ethics*. Belmont, CA: Wadsworth Publishing, 1992. Chapter 2.

Murray, Thomas H. and Arthur L. Caplan, eds. *Which Babies Shall Live?* Clifton, NJ: Humana Press, 1985.

Pence, Gregory E. *Classic Cases in Medical Ethics*. 2nd ed. New York: McGraw-Hill, 1995. Chapters 7 & 13.

_____. *Classic Works in Medical Ethics: Core Philosophical Readings*. New York: McGraw-Hill, 1998. Chapter 6.

Ramsey, Paul. *Ethics at the Edges of Life: Medical and Legal Intersections*. New Haven, CT: Yale University Press, 1978. Chapters 5 & 6.

Shelp, Earl E. *Born to Die? Deciding the Fate of Critically Ill Newborns*. New York: Free Press, 1986.

Sparks, Richard C. *To Treat or Not to Treat: Bioethics and the Handicapped Newborn*. Mahwah, NJ: Paulist Press, 1988.

Tooley, Michael. *Abortion and Infanticide*. New York: Oxford University Press, 1983.

Wekesser, Carol, ed. *Euthanasia: Opposing Viewpoints*. San Diego: Greenhaven Press, 1995. Chapter 5.

Websites for Imperiled Newborns (There are very few sites dedicated to just imperiled newborns and infanticide. Several of the sites in the preceding chapters will contain information in this area as well.)

The Anencephalic: A Suitable Donor (http://www.asfhelp.com/cem/ Videopr.htm) This is actually a summary of a video debate on the use of anenecephalics as donors. The tape is for sale if you wish to purchase it, but the summary has some good soundbites arguing both sides.

The Infanticide/Abortion Link — the Dehumanization of Infants (http:// www.gargaro.com/infanticide.html) Interesting article written against infanticide.

Infanticide for Beginners (http://www.firstthings.com/ftissues/ft9801/ nuechterlein.html) An article originally published in the journal *First Things* about the rhetoric concerning infanticide.

Ohio Right to Life (http://www.ohiolife.org/) A good pro-life website with a separate page on infanticide.

Should we change our minds about infanticide? (http://www.discovery.org/ chapman/infants.html) An article written to protest infanticide.

Vital Signs Ministry (http://www.vitalsignsministries.org) A general pro-life ministry that has a number of items dealing with infanticide.

CHAPTER 6
Made, Not Begotten: Genetic Ethics

Made, Not Begotten: Genetic Ethics

Introduction
A. Genetics 101
B. Genetic Screening
  1. Four Types of Screening
    a. Neonatal Screening
    b. Prenatal Diagnosis
    c. Carrier Screening
    d. Predictive or Presymptomatic Screening
  2. Ethical Issues in Genetic Screening
    a. The Problem of Knowledge
    b. Confidentiality
    c. Mandatory Genetic Screening
C. Genetic Intervention
  1. Introduction
  2. General Ethical Issues in Genetic Intervention
  3. Specific Ethical Issues in Genetic Intervention
D. Genetic Research and Experimentation
  1. The Human Genome Project
  2. Cloning
  3 Conclusion

6

Consider the work of God,
For who is able to straighten what He has bent?
Ecclesiastes 7:13, NASB

The time is the "not too distant future." In a moment of reckless passion Marie and Antonio Freeman conceive a son. The voice of Vincent Freeman is heard, "They used to say that a child conceived in love is a child of happiness. They don't say that any more." At the moment of birth a blood sample is taken and placed in a machine that can immediately read the child's DNA. A nurse calls out the figures, "Neurological condition, 60% probability; Manic depression, 42% probability; ADD [Attention Deficit Disorder] 89% probability; Heart Disorder . . ." She pauses and looks at the physician, "99% probability." The nurse continues, "Early fatal potential. Life expectancy — 30.2 years." We see the look of despair on Antonio's face. The doctor asks them for the child's name and Marie answers "Anton . . ." but is interrupted by her husband, "No. . . . Vincent . . . Vincent Anton . . . ." We hear the voice of Vincent again, "Ten fingers and ten toes. That's all that used to matter. Not now. Now only seconds old, the exact time and cause of my death was already known."

Later, Vincent's parents decide to have another child. This time they choose the "natural way." This son is genetically engineered. The parents come to the local geneticist's office for an interview. The geneticist explains what they have done so far. They extracted several eggs from Marie and fertilized them *in vitro*. After screening the eggs they end up with two healthy boys and two healthy girls. He informs them that there are no critical dispositions for major diseases and says that they need to select the gender, eyes, hair and skin color. Marie and Antonio respond that they would like a brother for Vincent. The geneticist goes on and explains that they will eradicate any potentially prejudicial conditions: premature baldness, myopia, alcoholism addictive susceptibility, propensity for violence, and obesity. The parents interrupt asking if, perhaps, just some things could be left to chance. The geneticist explains, "You want to give your child the best possible start. Believe me, we have enough imperfection built in already. Your child doesn't need any additional burdens. And keep in mind, this child is still you — it's simply the best of you. You could conceive naturally a thousand times and never get such a result." When the child is born he is named Anton, the voice of Vincent telling us "a child worthy of my father's name."

As they grow, Anton excels in every area and becomes the favorite son. Vincent's DNA follows him throughout his life. We observe how, as a child, he is denied admission to school because of his "chronic illness" and how the school's insurance won't cover him. As a teenager, he dreams of becoming an astronaut. His mother discourages him, telling him to be realistic. His chances are one in a hundred of being accepted into the program with his "heart condition." As an adult, we see how, at each job interview, a "drug screen" is performed. Vincent's voice tells us that everyone knows what they are really checking — DNA. There is a law against such discrimination, called Genoism, but it is a law no one takes seriously. If you refuse to disclose, they can take a sample from secretions left by your hand off a door handle, or a handshake, or the sweat left on the application you turn in. Vincent tells us that it is a world where they have "discrimination down to a science." There is now a new underclass, "In-valids." These are people discriminated against not because of race or religion, but because of "inferior" DNA. To the in-valids are left the menial and unimportant tasks in society while the "valids," the genetically engineered elite, are given the better jobs and the better lives.

It is a different world than the one we know. It is the world of *Gattaca*.[1]

Genetics 101   Is a world like that portrayed in the 1997 film *Gattaca* possible? While we do not have the technology to be there yet, the progress we have made in genetic research in the past few decades indicates that we are not far from at least the possibility of a society much like the one Vincent Freeman lives in. While the advances in **genetic screening**, therapy and engineering promise great benefits in solving genetic disorders and diseases, they also raise disturbing questions: Will we be forced to undergo genetic screening? Who will be able to obtain our genetic information? What about genetic discrimination? How easy will it be to shift from *treatment for* the human race to *enhancement of* the human race?

In order to understand the ethical issues behind the different aspects of genetic research we need to understand a little about genetics. Certainly one of the most important discoveries of this century was the 1953 discovery by two scientists,

James D. Watson and Francis Crick, of the basic structure of the DNA (deoxyribonucleic acid) molecule. This is the famous "double-helix" model that looks like a spiraling staircase. DNA is responsible for transmitting hereditary characteristics from parent to child. Watson and Crick's discovery laid the groundwork for understanding the basic mechanism for copying genetic material from one cell to another and from one human generation to another. This would eventually lead to recombinant DNA research, screening of genetic diseases, gene therapy and mapping the entire human genome.

> *One of the most important discoveries of this century was the 1953 discovery of the basic structure of the DNA molecule.*

We need to begin by distinguishing between cells, genes, and chromosomes. A *cell* is the basic unit of life. The human body is a living system of several trillion cells. Millions of these cells die off and are replaced by new ones every day. Some last longer than others and some, like brain cells, are not replaceable at all. We have different kinds of cells that perform different functions — liver cells, brain cells, etc. Inside each cell is a nucleus, and in the nucleus are tiny strands called *chromosomes*. Each cell nucleus contains 46 chromosomes in 23 pairs (except the reproductive cells which we will discuss below). Chromosomes are long strands made up of DNA and other chemicals. A *gene* is a section of DNA and is the basic physical and functional unit of heredity. A gene is a specific sequence of nucleotide bases. These sequences are instructions required for constructing proteins. Proteins provide the structural components for cells, tissues, and enzymes necessary for the essential biochemical reactions for all living things.

The British biologist, Richard Dawkins, provided a well known analogy to understand how this is all put together.[2]

Dawkins compared the human body to a library building containing many rooms. Each room represents a cell, so there are many trillions of rooms. In each room there is a bookcase (nucleus) that contains the architect's plan for the entire building.[3] The plans are located in 46 volumes (chromosomes). Each volume contains about 100,000 pages of information (genes) and each page contains 3 to 3.5 billion words (DNA molecules). The letters that compose the words on each page, the alphabet used by the architect, begin with the combinations of only four nucleic acids. These acids are paired up together in "base pairs" and combine in different orders to make up different sequences. There are about 3-3.5 billion base pairs in each gene. Like letters in a word, and words in a sentence, the sequence determines the "meaning" of the instructions given in the blueprint. If the instructions say one thing in one room, they will say the same thing in every room. Sometimes these instructions give incorrect information, and when that occurs we have genetic disorders and diseases.

How is all this passed down from parent to child? As we said, every cell in the body has 46 chromosomes, except the reproductive cells. Sperm and eggs each have 23 chromosomes. The genetic combinations of each sperm and each egg is different and unique. In fact, it is estimated that each parent is capable of producing more than 19 trillion different combinations of genes, explaining why there is so much variety even between members of the same family. This variety is compounded even more through the process known as *meiosis*. This has to do with the developing of the reproductive cells.

During the making of a sperm or egg, pieces of each chromosome inherited from an individual's father change places with matching chromosomes from his mother. To understand this, let's return to Dawkins library illustration.[4] We said that each bookcase contains 46 volumes (chromosomes). To be precise, the 46 volumes are not 46 different volumes, but are actually 23 matched volumes. These volumes are like loose-leaf binders. During meiosis, pages (genes) from one volume are swapped with those from an exactly matching volume.

This is called recombination. This results in a mixing up of bits of the 46 volumes. The 23 volumes in the reproductive genes are a combination of different pages from all 46 master volumes.

At fertilization the 23 chromosomes of one parent become paired with 23 chromosomes of the other parent, and a brand new set of 46 chromosomes comes into existence. To use our library analogy, a brand new blueprint guiding the building and developing of a brand new library building now exists. The primary reason this new library is so different from the old one is the process of recombination. It is not that new genes exist, it is just a new combination of the old genes.

There are two other distinctions that need to be addressed to understand genetics. First, the cells that become sperm and egg are called *germ cells* because they contain information that will be passed on to further generations. All the other cells in our body are called *somatic cells*. Nothing in somatic cells is passed on to future generations, and any change in them will only affect the person of whom they are a part. This distinction will become important when we discuss **genetic intervention** and therapy.

The cells that become sperm and egg are called germ cells; all other cells are called somatic cells.

The second distinction is between *recessive* and *dominant* genes. Dominant genes are "expressed," and recessive genes are usually "unexpressed." If no dominant gene is present, then the recessive gene will express itself. However, a dominant gene will always eclipse a recessive gene. To use our library illustration, think of some pages in one volume as rough drafts (recessive genes) and the matching pages in the matching volume as final drafts (dominant genes). The blueprint will always refer to the final draft.[5] For example, suppose someone has a particular dominant gene, like the gene for brown eyes is said to be, and has a recessive gene, like the gene for blue eyes. The result is that the person will have brown eyes. However, what if one has two rough drafts (recessive genes)? The two rough drafts of the page will come together and be accepted as the final draft. If one has two recessive blue-eyed genes, he or she will have blue eyes.

Finally, if one has a recessive gene, that gene may not be expressed, but it can still be passed on to other generations. In other words, during meiosis, when the "pages" are getting mixed together, some of the rough drafts may get mixed into the 23 reproductive chromosomes. Therefore, if one has a recessive blue-eyed gene and a dominant brown-eyed gene, he will have brown eyes, but will have a 50% chance of passing on his blue-eyed gene. Whether his offspring has blue eyes or not will depend on the genes of its mother. This is important for understanding the passing on of certain genetic disorders. One may not have a particular disorder, but could be a *carrier* of the disease.

> *One may not have a particular disorder, but could be a carrier of the disease.*

Sometimes, the process of passing on genes goes wrong and genetic disorders occur. John Fletcher lists five main reasons this can happen.[6] First, there can be the presence of *chromosomal abnormalities*. The chromosomes of the sperm and egg are abnormal before fertilization ever occurs. They can be defective, missing something, stick together or break apart abnormally. Second, there may have been an *abnormal process of cell division*. This will result in too many or too few chromosomes. The most common form of this is when the cell fails to divide properly on chromosome number 21. The result is three chromosomes instead of two, hence Trisomy 21, which is Down's syndrome. Third, there is the possibility of an *inborn error of metabolism*. A gene sends the wrong message, and results in a biological defect. This defect is usually a defi-

ciency or abnormal accumulation of certain necessary substances. These kinds of genetic conditions are often found in
ethnic groups who experience specific genetic disorders, such
as sickle-cell disease among African-Americans or Tay-Sachs
disease among those of Ashkenazi Jewish descent. A fourth
reason for genetic disorders are *mutations* in the genes. These
are often random and we don't always understand why they
occur. For example, radiation exposure can cause a mutation
on the genetic level. Once the gene is changed, all the harm,
or sometimes the benefit, is copied to every other cell. Finally,
Fletcher lists that there are *multifactorial* reasons for genetic
disorders. This is a combination of any of the above plus environmental factors.

According to one source, in the latest catalog of genetic
disorders there are described 5,710 distinguishable genetic or
chromosomal conditions.[7] Statistically, genetic disorders are
the second leading cause of death among children aged 1-4 in
the United States and the third leading cause of death among
teenagers 15-17. Twenty-five to thirty percent of admissions
to hospitals in the United States for children under 18, and
13% of adults are estimated to be due to genetic disorders.
Also, 20-25% of institutionalized mentally retarded persons
have genetic disorders.[8]

There are a number of different activities geneticists are
involved with to help solve the problems of genetic disorders.
In this chapter we will divide them into three areas: genetic
screening, genetic intervention, and genetic research and
experimentation. In each area, we will first describe the current practices and activities and then discuss some of the ethical problems and issues relating to that area.

Genetic Screening

The major advances in genetics have been in the areas of
diagnosis and prediction of genetic disorders. We can presently
diagnose far more than we can treat. These activities involve
genetic screening. Leroy Walters defines a genetic test as "the
use of diagnostic procedures for determination of the presence
or absence of one or more genetic traits or conditions in an
individual."[9] There are four different kinds of screening.

1. *Neonatal screening.* This is genetically testing newborns for certain disorders and was the first form of genetic screening to come about. In the early 1960s a genetic test was developed by Dr. Robert Guthrie to test for PKU, an inborn error of metabolism that prevents the breakdown of phenylalanine, an amino acid. One result of this disorder is severe retardation. However, if discovered early, treatment is relatively simple by placing the infant on a diet very low in phenylalanine. The test consists of gaining a blood sample through a heel prick on the infant at birth. In 1963 Massachusetts became the first state to require the PKU screening for newborns. Today every state in the country has mandatory PKU screening.

> ## *Neonatal screening was the first form of genetic screening to come about.*

Since the 1960s mandatory neonatal testing for other diseases has included hypothyroidism, sickle-cell anemia, galactosemia, homocystinuria and maple-syrup urine disease.[10] Screening for other conditions such as cystic fibrosis, heart disease and HIV are under discussion. Only a handful of states allow for the refusal of newborn screening, usually on religious grounds.

2. *Prenatal Diagnosis.* This is the genetic testing of a fetus. It was historically the second type of genetic testing to develop. In 1966 the first study of cells drawn from the amniotic sac by a process known as *amniocentesis* was performed. Over the following two years successful diagnosis of a chromosomal abnormality and diagnosis of an inborn error of metabolism occurred. Today, along with amniocentesis, a number of prenatal genetic tests are performed and include the following: (1) Maternal serum alpha feto protein (MSAFP) screening, a blood test of the mother usually performed between 16-18 weeks of pregnancy that can predict high

chances of a spina bifida or anencephalic child; (2) Enhanced MSAFP, sometimes referred to as a "downscreen" because of its ability (60-65% accuracy) to predict babies with Down's syndrome; (3) Chorionic Villus Sampling (CVS), a rare and risky test used for chromosomal analysis and DNA study, where a piece of the chorion, or outer tissue of the amniotic sac, is removed for testing. The chances for fetal damage and miscarriage as a result of this test is high; (4) Percutaneous Umbilical Blood Sampling (PUBS), a newer and even riskier genetic test in which blood is taken from the umbilical cord of a fetus to measure blood components and determine if there are fetal/maternal blood conflicts; and (5) Fetal Biopsy which is used to obtain skin samples to perform DNA tests.

Today prenatal testing can diagnose over one hundred genetic disorders including Tay-Sachs Disease, Down's syndrome, Cystic Fibrosis, Spina Bifida, Trisomy 13, Trisomy 18, Sickle-Cell Anemia, Muscular Dystrophy and Hemophilia. In addition to standard prenatal testing, a new form of testing on embryos fertilized *in vitro*[11] has evolved, called preimplantation diagnosis. After fertilization, the cells of the zygote begin to divide. When it reaches the 4-8-cell stage, one cell is removed for testing and the other cells are cryogenically frozen. The cell is tested for a host of genetic diseases. If it is healthy the other cells are unfrozen and implanted in the womb. If it is not healthy, the cells are discarded. This test is particularly useful for detecting early development of genetic disorders. It is still in an experimental stage and is usually only performed on those using assisted forms of reproduction, though parents who are not in need of assisted reproduction may make use of *in vitro* if they want an early embryonic genetic test.

3. *Carrier Screening.* Above we commented that it is possible not to have a genetic disorder, but to be a carrier of one if it is on a recessive gene. This type of genetic screening is usually done when one desires to know if he or she will pass on a genetic disorder to his or her children. Most often couples will consider such a screening if they are contemplating marriage. Carrier screening almost always is performed only on those

who have a suspicion that they might be carriers of genetic disorders. The most common groups tested as carriers are certain ethnic groups who have a higher than usual chance of a particular genetic disorder. For example, Tay-Sachs disease primarily affects Ashkenazi (eastern European) Jewish descendants though it is also prevalent among French Canadians. Sickle-cell anemia is prevalent among Africans and African-Americans. Mediterraneans and Southeast Asians are susceptible to thalassemia, a hemoglobin disorder similar to sickle-cell anemia. Some genetic diseases are family or gender related, and individuals who have a family history of certain disorders might want to be tested to determine if they are carriers.

Although most carrier testing is voluntary, there have been moves to require such testing.

Most carrier testing is voluntary, but there have been moves in the past to require such testing. In 1970 a relatively inexpensive test was developed for sickle-cell anemia making it possible to identify carriers of the disease. During 1971 and 1972 twelve states passed mandatory laws for testing African-Americans to determine if they were sickle-cell carriers as a condition to getting married. While the sickle-cell gene is dominant, the disease only occurs when both parents pass it on to their offspring. If two carriers marry, there is a chance of one out of four of their children contracting the disease. The laws did not forbid carriers to marry, but required they receive genetic counseling. Soon employers and insurance companies began to require the tests. Charges of discrimination and even genocide of the African-American population were made. In 1972 Congress stepped in and passed the National Sickle-Cell Anemia Control Act, forcing states that received federal funds to make sickle-cell screening voluntary. In 1976 the National Genetic Disease Act was passed and provided funding for testing and genetic counseling, reinforcing the voluntary aspect of these programs.

Couples who go through carrier testing usually receive genetic counseling. The counselor will obtain cell samples from the couple, analyze them for genetic disorders, and then help the couple to understand the risks involved in having a child who would either have the disease or be a carrier. If it is a recessive trait, and only one member of the couple carries it, then they will not produce a child with the disease, but their chances are 50-50 for producing a carrier. If both members have the recessive genetic disorder, their chances are 25% of producing a child with that disorder, 25% of not producing a child with it, and 50-50 of producing a carrier. For some couples such information may be important for choosing a mate and deciding to have children.

An example can be found among a tight Orthodox Jewish community in New York City. They have developed a program called Dor Yeshorim ("the generation of the righteous"). Within the community teenagers are tested for their carrier status of Tay-Sachs disease, which has been especially prevalent among this community. This information, encoded with identification numbers for confidentiality purposes, is kept in a central office. When a boy and girl want to seriously date, they are encouraged to check with the office to determine their status as carriers. If there is a significant risk of having a child with the genetic disease, they are discouraged from a serious relationship. The program has been successful in significantly reducing the number of Tay-Sachs cases within the community.

4. *Predictive or Presymptomatic Screening*. This fourth type of genetic testing is the most recent and will probably expand over the next decade. It allows persons with family histories of certain genetic disorders to be tested to see if they are at risk of developing the disorder. It is called "presymptomatic" because the test is taken long before any symptoms of the genetic disorder might develop. A common genetic disorder that falls under this test is Huntington's disease.

Huntington's disease (HD) strikes a person later in life, usually between 35 to 45 years of age. The person gradually deteriorates over a 10- to 20-year period as he or she loses motor functions and cognitive abilities. At present, there is no cure for the disease and it is always fatal. In 1983 a "marker" for HD was found. A marker can be used in developing linkage tests to help locate the gene itself. Linkage tests require blood samples from several generations of a family and a comprehensive family background is needed. Even then, the linkage test may not be completely accurate, because the marker didn't always travel with the gene. The linkage test became available in May 1987, and was offered through three medical centers in the United States. However, turnout was very low. Of the estimated 1,500 people at risk in the New England area, only 32 signed up for the preliminary counseling, and only 18 actually took the test.[12] In 1993 the actual HD gene was finally discovered. Now persons from families with a history of HD can be tested for HD.

Once we have knowledge of defects, what can we do about it?

Since the discovery of the HD marker and subsequent gene, a number of other genes responsible for genetic disorders have been discovered, including early-onset Alzheimer's, hemochromatosis, polycystic kidney disease, family-inherited hypercholesterolemia, and some genetic forms of cancers. All of these can be tested for presymptomatically. In addition a new area has developed called *ecogenetics*, which studies situations in which it is not just the gene that causes the disorder but a combination of the genetic and environmental agents that are encountered. One discovery is a particular gene on chromosome 15 that turns cigarette smoke into carcinogens, but will do nothing if cigarette smoke is not introduced into a person's system.[13]

Ethical Issues in Genetic Screening

1. *The Problem of Knowledge.* One of the primary questions that arises out of genetic screening is: Once we have this

knowledge, what can we do about it? The 1983 President's Commission on Bioethics reached the following conclusion about genetic screening:

> In sum, the fundamental value of genetic screening and counseling is their ability to enhance the opportunities for individuals to obtain information about their personal health and make autonomous choices based on that information.[14]

However, at present only a handful of genetic diseases are treatable, and therefore advance knowledge can do nothing to prevent the onset of the disease nor treat it once it begins. Therefore one is not sure what "autonomous choices" one can make. Having knowledge of most genetic diseases just doesn't seem to help very much and, in fact, it may be harmful.

For example, take prenatal and preimplantation screening. Such screening is done to determine if a fetus has a specific genetic disorder, and has become almost routine in pregnancy. We have had three children, and in every case my wife was approached about having the MSAFP test (she refused each time). If the test comes back positive, what is the parent supposed to do? The most common answer is to abort the fetus, for that is the only way to "treat" the disease. Christian philosopher Scott Rae calls this "the abortion assumption" and comments how, for some, this assumption underlies the whole purpose of prenatal screening:

> Most genetic counsellors will say that they operate with the presumption of objectivity. Their role is to give information and maximize reproductive choice for the couple. Yet when public health officials talk about the benefits of prenatal screening in reducing the incidence of genetic diseases, they typically assume that couples will end their pregnancy if they receive bad news from their testing. . . . Public health authorities sometimes suggest that prenatal testing is a great help in eliminating the incidence of genetic disease. But the only way it can be helpful in that way is if couples end their pregnancies. The genetic disease is thereby eliminated, but at the expense of the child who has the disease.[15]

We have already discussed the issue of abortion and infanticide decisions based on quality-of-life arguments in previous chapters and therefore will only make a few comments here. First, and most important, the fetus, by nature of the kind of being it is, is a human person from the moment of conception. The presence of a genetic disorder does not in any way diminish its personhood. As a human person, it is an image-of-God-bearer and therefore to take its life is an affront to God himself. In fact, the genetically impaired fetus is as much a human person as a genetically impaired adult and no one advocates killing adults with genetic disorders (at least not yet).

Second, genetic tests are not completely accurate. Many of them have substantial margins of error for false positives and false negatives. For example, the enhanced MSAFP test has only a 60%-65% accuracy for detecting Down's syndrome which is the primary disorder it is designed to detect. The regular AFP is *designed* to create a number of false positives which then have to be confirmed by further testing causing tremendous anxiety to the parents. It would be unwise to make a decision to take the life of a child based upon such tests.

Many genetic tests have substantial margins of error for false positives and false negatives.

Third, even if such tests are accurate, they cannot inform one of the magnitude of deformity. For several genetic disorders there are differing degrees of abnormality. A Down's syndrome child can range from mild retardation to very severe cases, and prenatal testing cannot inform anyone where a child will fit in that continuum.

Fourth, it is simply discriminatory and presumptuous to say that a person with genetic disorders has no right to life. Right to life is something all persons have regardless of their genes. Also, no one can arbitrarily make that decision for another person. We explained in the previous chapter how difficult it is to arrive at a "best interests view" for an infant.

Finally, there is the possibility that one might not be thinking only in terms of the burdens on the infant. Scott Rae comments:

> Not even parents should have the right to set the standard of a 'life worth living' for their child. It is all too easy for the parents to confuse the burden of life for the child with the burden on the parents of caring for the child. The notion of a life not worth living should not be used to disguise the wish of parents to avoid a great burden themselves.[16]

One can see this discrimination most clearly when one looks at the guidelines suggested by the 1983 President's Council on Bioethics. In no uncertain terms they make it clear that it would be inappropriate and immoral to use genetic screening for sex selection. This is because most couples seem to want male children, which would make such screening discriminatory against women. However, using genetic screening for genetic disorders in order to eliminate the disorders (which can only be done through abortion) is just as discriminatory — it's just not recognized as such. This is really a form of **eugenics** called negative eugenics. We will discuss eugenics more below.

All of these problems with prenatal screening have led some to suggest that it is inappropriate altogether. Christian ethicist Gilbert Meilaender holds such a view. He comments how love is the most important of the Christian virtues and quotes Josef Pieper's definition of love as a way of saying to another: "It's good that you exist; it's good that you are in this world!"[17] Meilaender goes on to say:

> Precisely because we know ourselves to have been loved this unqualifiedly by God, and because we know we should learn to love others as we have been loved, Christians ought to set themselves against any prenatal screening, at least as it is currently practiced in this country in an increasingly routinized way. For it stands in conflict with the virtue that would say to another: "It's good that you exist."[18]

Meilaender also points out that prenatal screening, followed by abortion, changes the whole relationship between mother and child. The relationship becomes more tentative and conditional because the mother is free to "walk away" from the child if she feels the child is too much of a burden. However, with such freedom comes responsibility: the responsibility to be tested if one is suspicious, the responsibility of making a choice, and the responsibility of the consequences of that choice. He suggests that we might begin to see lawsuits brought against mothers who did not abort their genetically disordered children by the children themselves who feel they should have been aborted rather than live a life that is "worse than nonexistence." With knowledge comes power and responsibility. We are "playing God" in a very real sense. Our children may turn to us, like Job, asking us, "Why did you allow this evil to happen when you had the knowledge and means to prevent it?" Meilaender believes that such a responsibility is too great for us to bear. We were never meant to — it is God's alone.

> *We were never meant to bear such a responsibility — it is God's alone.*

Not everyone agrees with Meilaender's rejection of prenatal screening. Scott Rae believes that tests with little risk can be valuable in preparing parents "for the emotional and perhaps financial rigors of raising a handicapped child."[19] Meilaender, however, believes that parents are deceiving themselves if they believe that such screening will help prepare them for the child: "It does exactly the opposite. It sets our foot on a path that is difficult to exit. . . . It prepares us not for the kind of commitment that parenthood requires, an unconditional commitment, but for a kind of responsibility that finite beings ought to reject."[20] While prenatal screening is not wrong *per se*, couples need to ask themselves what they plan to do with the knowledge they gain through screening, and what that screening might be saying about themselves and their commitment to their child.

Prenatal screening is not the only area where the question of what to do with the knowledge of a genetic disorder arises. It is also problematic for other types of screening. If an infant undergoes a neonatal screen that determines that he will develop Tay-Sachs disease or muscular dystrophy, that could possibly lead parents to treat him differently, like Vincent was treated in the story of *Gattaca*. If they know the infant will not live long, they may not give him the love and attention he deserves and needs because they do no want to make such an "investment" in something that will not last long or go far. They may even consider neonaticide rather than having to care for children that will die or suffer at a very young age. They would just have to find a doctor sympathetic to such a view.

Carrier screening that allows people to know they are carrying a genetic flaw also raises some tough ethical alternatives. If they have knowledge that they may pass on a genetic disorder, do they have a moral obligation not to get married or, if they do marry, not to have children? Should they seek sterilization even though screening might not be accurate or the chances are only one in four?

Should a possible carrier seek sterilization even though screening might not be accurate or the chances of transmission slim?

Presymptomatic screening and knowledge also raise a difficult issue. Is it better to know for sure if you do or don't have a genetic disorder, or is it better not to know? Suppose a person is suspicious that she might have HD and so she is tested for it and finds out that she will develop the disease. How might that affect her life? She might decide that she cannot be happy living any more and opt for an early assisted suicide. Should she be given that option? Over 25% of HD victims consider suicide and 10% actually carry it out.[21] How much higher might that go as more are tested for the disease? Many of those who don't commit suicide take on a "sick identity" in which they dramatically alter their lives and take on the role of being ill, including depression, anxiety, and hypochondria, even though they are currently perfectly healthy.

2. *Confidentiality*. Closely related to the question of knowledge is the question of who else will be able to access the knowledge of a genetic disorder. Normally, health information is kept confidential between physician and patient. However, others may believe they have a right to your genetic information. This is problematic in a number of contexts.

a. *Family*. Most people will probably volunteer information to other family members if it concerns health-related issues. But it is possible that someone might not wish to disclose that information to other family members for a number of reasons. However, if he doesn't disclose, does the physician have a duty to disclose to other family members if he believes that by not disclosing he is putting those family members in danger? Suppose Harry is tested and finds out he has the gene for HD. Since HD is a dominant gene, inheriting it from either parent will lead to the disease. Harry has a 50% chance of passing it to his children and they would have the same chance of passing it on to their children. Does Harry have a moral obligation to disclose? Suppose he refuses to disclose his condition to his children. Does Harry's doctor now have an obligation to break confidence and tell them? One must consider, in reflecting on these questions, such things as: the importance of physician/ patient confidentiality, the fact that there is only a 50% chance of children getting the gene, and the question we discussed above of what good the knowledge will be to them. Disclosing might be more harmful than helpful.

b. *Medical insurance*. Insurance companies argue that they have a right to this information. After all, they have a legitimate interest in controlling costs and therefore want to insure persons who are at low risk of disease or debilitation. If they get your genetic information and find there is a 60% chance of your developing a genetic heart disorder, they might charge a higher premium or even refuse to insure you, even though you might be perfectly healthy and never actually develop the disease. One legislative move to confront this problem was the passage of the Health Insurance Portability and Accountability Act of 1996 which prohibits insurance discrimination on the basis of genetics.

c. *Employment*. Think back to the story of *Gattaca*. Businesses may feel they have a right to your genetic screen. Like insurance companies, businesses have a legitimate interest to control costs, and they may not want to invest in hiring and training an employee if they know he might become ill early in life. However, this constitutes discrimination. It's not even discrimination on the basis of handicap, but on a *possible future* handicap. While the Equal Employment Opportunities Commission has ruled denial of jobs on the basis of genetic information is illegal, many argue that there are still too many loopholes and exceptions.

d. *Government*. If a person has a genetic disorder, there is a good possibility that he or she will eventually need state or federal resources to help defray medical costs. Therefore, the government might want to know a person's genetic screen. We mentioned above the Sickle-Cell Laws of the early 1970s. These were enacted by state governments and required that African-Americans be tested for the sickle-cell trait before getting married. The idea was that by knowing their status in relation to sickle-cell, married couples could think through their options and plans for children. However, as a result of the laws, many African-Americans lost their jobs, health insurance, and were even discharged from the military even though they were perfectly healthy and with no risk of developing the disease.[22]

All four of these contexts raise the issue of confidentiality in genetic testing and the danger of discrimination. In one study in the New England area, 41 separate incidents of discrimination were reported. Thirty-two of these were insurance incidents and 7 were employment related.[23] Doctor Christopher Hook commenting on this study reports,

> Many of the individuals involved had undergone testing only because another family member had been affected with a genetic condition; they themselves were still healthy. One patient with a heredity hemochromatosis, a disease of iron absorption and storage which can be well managed, was denied insurance. He stated: "I might as well have had AIDS." Another case involved the brother of an individual who had Gaucher's disease. This brother was screened and the results suggested that he was an asymptomatic carrier. When he applied for a governmental job and included the history of his testing in the application, he was denied the job because he was "a carrier like sickle cell."[24]

A 1996 Harvard/Stanford University study documented 206 cases of genetic discrimination by "businesses, insurance companies, schools, blood banks and the military. Included among the cases was a situation in which a woman's HMO would pay for an abortion of the woman's fetus that carried a gene for cystic fibrosis, but would not pay for the birth and care of the child if it were born."[25]

In today's medical world, complete confidentiality is extremely difficult to maintain.

In today's medical world, complete confidentiality is extremely difficult to maintain. There are just too many people who need access to patient records. Physicians, nurses, hospital personnel, billing personnel, insurance companies, and HMOs are just some of the many people who may have access to a person's genetic screen. So far little has been proposed to rectify the problem. Breaching confidentiality may sometimes be necessary, but in every case strong evidence must be presented to justify the breach.

3. *Mandatory Genetic Screening*. The issue of mandatory screening is closely related to the above issue. If there are those who believe they have a right to your genetic screen, there is a good chance they may *require* you to undergo screening. Currently, all prenatal screening and presymptomatic screening is voluntary. While some forms of carrier screening were mandated years ago, no such laws are present today. However, some experts fear that some prenatal screening could become mandatory in the years ahead. Once it is determined that there is a social issue demanding fetal genetic knowledge, states and the federal government may pass laws deciding that social need trumps individual liberty. This is precisely how many laws in our country have evolved.

At the state level a number of newborn screening tests are mandatory. The most common of these is the PKU screening. These mandatory laws are justified on a number of grounds. PKU is treatable by diet, but treatment must begin right away. Therefore a neonatal screen is justifiable. The PKU test is a very low risk test, requiring only a heel prick blood sample. Very few people see PKU as coercive, and in fact are generally thankful for the test. However, some are concerned that blanket "acceptance" of current mandatory laws may encourage the passing of other mandatory laws. In recent years states have expanded the mandatory newborn screening laws for other genetic diseases. It is questionable whether these laws are as easily justified.

While the government has so far required little more than newborn screening, the private sector has not been as dormant. Both insurance companies and employers have attempted to require genetic screening in order to obtain insurance or employment. Carol Haas writes, "Some employers are advocating that applicants and employees be genetically screened to determine whether they have a predisposition to contracting occupational disorders. Such screening hasn't caught on in popularity, mainly because the technology is still unsophisticated, unreliable, and very expensive. But it may only be a matter of time until employees are told, whether they want to be or not, that they are susceptible to certain diseases."[26]

It may only be a matter of time until employees are told, whether they want to be or not, that they are susceptible to certain diseases.

A recent case shows how screening is a current problem in the workplace. While this is not a case of mandatory *genetic* testing, it does demonstrate how close we are to such testing The case is *Norman-Bloodsaw v. Lawrence* and it was argued on June 10, 1997, in the 9th Circuit Court of Appeals. The case concerns a number of administrative and clerical employees of Lawrence Berkeley Laboratory, a research facility operated by the University of California. The employees, headed by Marya S. Norman-Bloodsaw, alleged that, in the course of their mandatory preemployment entrance health exams and on subsequent occasions, Lawrence Berkeley Laboratory tested their blood and urine for syphilis, pregnancy, and sickle-cell trait without their knowledge or consent and without subsequently informing employees of the test results. Upon being hired, the employees agreed to fill out a health evaluation questionnaire and undergo a health examination which included the providing of blood and urine samples. While the evaluation form asked the employees if they had any history of sickle-cell anemia, venereal disease or menstrual disorders, nothing was said or implied that they would be tested for any of these diseases. Health evaluations are not uncommon for many corporations, and they often include standard blood tests and drug screens. However, as several experts testified in the district court hearing:

> The manner in which the tests were performed was inconsistent with sound medical practice . . . medical scholars roundly condemn[ed] Lawrence's alleged practices and explain[ed], *inter alia*, that testing for syphilis, sickle-cell trait,

and pregnancy is not an appropriate part of an occupational medical examination and is rarely if ever done by employers as a matter of routine.[27]

The employees sued the laboratory on the basis of the Americans with Disabilities Act (requiring medical testing that was not job related), Title VII of the Civil Rights Act of 1964 (discrimination against African-Americans in testing for the sickle-cell trait), and their right to privacy as guaranteed by both the United Sates Constitution and the California State Constitution (testing without gaining informed consent). However, the district court summarily dismissed the case holding that (1) the statute of limitations had run out on all three of the above claims and (2) the fact that tests were "part of a comprehensive medical examination to which the plaintiffs consented." Therefore, the district court concluded that there were "sufficient facts to put them [the employees] on notice" and they should have expected the testing. The case was appealed to the 9th Circuit Court of Appeals who reversed the lower court's ruling on the Title VII claims and right to privacy claims. They ruled that (1) the statute of limitations had not run out on any of these claims; (2) the lower court erred in not considering whether these tests were acceptable; that a trial was necessary to determine that issue; (3) these tests were not necessary, were an invasion of privacy, and the sickle-cell tests were discriminatory.

Whether or not government or private mandatory genetic screening will come about is still open to debate. Currently, most are leaning toward a voluntary approach. However, there are those who argue that with such freedom comes responsibility and that one may have a moral duty, if not a legal one, to be tested for a genetic disorder or trait if one has reason to believe he or she is susceptible to a genetic disorder. LeRoy Walters argues that,

> Individuals and couples have a moral duty to learn what they can about the likelihood that they will transmit genetic conditions to their offspring and to take reasonable steps — steps that are compatible with their other ethical convictions — to avoid causing preventable harm to their descendants.[28]

Walters does not believe such an "ethics of genetic duty" should be legalized. However, the move from voluntary to required sometimes is not a large one and can be very subtle. Once a person is required to know, it is very easy to be required to do something about it.

Genetic Intervention   Genetic Intervention involves actually manipulating genes in order to improve them. This is sometimes called genetic engineering or genetic therapy. Genetic engineering actually takes place in other areas besides human health programs. Gene splicing or recombinant DNA technology has been useful in such areas as agriculture and environmental technology. New and healthier crops have been developed to help feed more people. Proteins have been developed that enhance animal health. On the environmental level, genetically altered bacteria have been developed that will feed on oil slicks to help clean up oil spills, and more is being done to develop ways of converting waste materials into useful products, such as organic wastes into sugar, alcohol and methane.

Genetic engineering has not been without its critics.

Such genetic engineering has not been without its critics and some have been leery about changing nature in such a fundamental way. Some argue that, if we are so easily going to allow gene splicing on the plant and animal level, can human gene splicing be far behind? Others are concerned about the commercialization of nature. In 1987 the U.S. Patent and Trademark office announced that all forms of animal life, with the exception of humans, should be considered "patentable" subject matter. All life can now be regarded as a manufacture or composition of matter.[29] With commercialization some believe that corporate profits may take priority over ethical behavior, or argue that genetic engineering may have disastrous effects on the environment. The possibility of biological weapons and germ warfare concerns most of us. A serious issue, which has not received enough attention, has to do with regulating genetic experimentation, especially in the private sector. All of these concerns should signal us that we need to approach the issue of genetic engineering very cautiously.

When genetic engineering is directed at humans, it is usually referred to as gene therapy. We stated earlier that genetic screening is the main activity taking place in genetics today. This is primarily due to the fact that our technology is still in its infancy when it comes to actually being able to intervene in a person's genetic makeup and make changes. However, it is the goal of almost all geneticists to be able to perform genetic engineering on human beings. What kind of intervention can or may be done someday?

There are four types of intervention that might someday become available.

In a well-known article, Nelson Wivel and Leroy Walters arrived at four types of intervention that might someday become available, and to a small degree some of this is currently taking place.[30] The four types occur by combining two factors. The first factor has to do with the distinction between somatic-cell therapy and **germ-line therapy**. Remembering what we said earlier in the chapter concerning the differences between somatic and germ cells will help in understanding this distinction. *Somatic-cell therapy* is intervention which aims to cure a genetic disorder by modifying the nonreproductive cells in a person. If successful, this would cure the person, but he would not pass that cure on to other generations. For example, experimental treatment is being attempted to modify the bone marrow cells of a person with sickle-cell anemia. The bone marrow is where red blood cells are manufactured; by modifying the cells one could eradicate the sickle-cell gene, thereby curing the person. However, she would not be able to pass this on to her children. *Germ-line therapy* is an intervention in the reproductive cells to attempt to modify them so that a particular genetic disorder would not be passed on to future generations. In this type of intervention both somatic cells and germ-line cells are treated to affect both the present person and her future offspring. There are obvious concerns with germ-line therapy that are not present with somatic-cell therapy.

The other factor involved with the different types of intervention concerns the distinction between therapy and enhancement. This line is not always obvious. *Therapy* has to do with the curing or preventing of a genetic disorder. We have already discussed a number of genetic disorders which almost all agree would be beneficial to cure: Huntington's Disease, Tay-Sachs, Down's syndrome, Sickle-cell Anemia, and many others. *Enhancement* has to do with improving traits and abilities that are not diseases. Improving one's intelligence, memory, lifespan, and physical capabilities are all examples of enhancement. Rather than curing, we are actually improving the person. Taking these two factors into consideration, there are four possible types of genetic intervention: somatic-cell therapy, germ-line cell therapy, somatic-cell enhancement, and germ-line cell enhancement.

The first successful somatic-cell therapy on a human person occurred on Sept. 14, 1990. Four-year-old Asahnti Dasilva had severe combined immune deficiency (SCID), a genetic disease that undermines the immune system, making it unable to fight diseases. Most who are born with this disorder die early from infection, usually before they are two. Geneticists at the National Institute of Health performed a procedure which involved removing T-cells (white blood cells), and inserting the proper gene into them to produce the immune enzyme. The T-cells then were reinjected into Asahnti's body to reproduce, spread throughout the system and produce the proper enzyme. It was not a cure, as the T-cells had to be replaced every couple of months, but Asahnti could now live a fairly normal life. Leroy Walters reports that by 1995, 99 additional somatic gene therapies have been reviewed and approved in the United States. Two-thirds are cancer-related, while others seek to cure cystic fibrosis, HIV, Gaucher's disease, and rheumatoid arthritis.[31]

As far as is known, germ-line therapy has not been performed on human beings. However, experiments have been performed on laboratory animals with some success. Genes have been inserted into early embryos of mice. As the embryos develop, the gene appears in the nucleus of each cell, including reproductive cells. When the mice later reproduce, the gene has been detected in their offspring. According to Walters, genetic defects have also been corrected in fruit flies and mice.[32] Germ-line therapy and somatic therapy are not always easily separated. Some genetic disorders need to be treated at the early embryonic stage in order to affect all the cells of the body. Since the reproductive cells will be included, one is doing somatic and germ-line therapy at the same time.

The only known enhancement studies occurred in 1982 in mice when they were given a gene for a growth hormone in early embryonic stages. Only a few mice made it to maturity, but a significant number were affected by the hormone and were substantially larger. When they produced offspring, the offspring were also significantly larger, demonstrating that the gene had been passed on to their young.

Ethical Issues in Genetic Intervention

Genetic intervention can offer many benefits. The possibility of curing, possibly forever, a number of genetic disorders is certainly an admirable and important goal in medical science. However, there are some very real concerns and moral problems with intervening in creation that should be a flashing yellow light, warning us to proceed with caution.

Two issues apply to any kind of genetic intervention. The first is the danger of commercialization. Many medical laboratories are run by large corporations. It would be naive to deny that one of the primary motivations behind genetic research is the possibility for enormous profits that a genetic cure would bring. Imagine the corporation that discovers and patents a cure for genetic heart disease or cystic fibrosis. The corporation would have complete control over the patent and could charge almost anything for it. Corporations can justify high prices by appealing to the expense of genetic research. Anticipation for profits might also cause companies to cut corners, place undue pressures on researchers, and slant studies in favor of the company. While there is some government regulation of genetic research itself, in a free-market society such as ours, it is difficult to see how government could regulate the distribution of genetic cures.

There is often an attitude in scientific research that says "If it can be done, then it should be done."

A second general issue is what I shall call the "scientific attitude." This is an attitude often present in the scientific community of running full speed ahead into scientific experimentation and research, without taking the time to think through the ethical and social issues that such knowledge and experimentation might affect. My point here is not to impugn science in general, nor any specific scientist. Those in medical science are often motivated by a desire to do good, to cure disease and make the world a better place for people to live. However, even pure motives can blind one to the social and ethical implications of scientific work. There is often an attitude in scientific research that says "If it *can* be done, then it *should* be done." Willard Gaylin, a bioethicist and founder of the Hastings Center, has said, "I not only think we should tamper with Mother Nature, I think Mother Nature wants us to."[33] In addition, science often has the attitude of "controlling" nature that often dominates scientific thinking. Evolutionary biologist Theodosius Dobzhansky states, "Evolution need no longer be a destiny imposed on us from without; it may be conceivably controlled by man, in accordance with his values and wisdom"[34] (which, of course, are merely products of evolution). Such attitudes can be dangerous if left without ethical and societal limits and controls. Charles Colson states it well: "So while genetic research may lead to important medical advances, we must probe the deeper question: What are the restraints? Technological advance may make it *possible* to do something, but *ought* we to do it?"[35] The restraints need to come from outside of science itself. These are not scientific issues; they are philosophical, ethical, societal and religious issues.

As far as specific types of interventions go, currently somatic-cell therapy is the only type that has been performed on human persons. Since this is therapeutic, few have been morally critical of it. There are those who believe that we should not be doing any genetic therapy at all. They argue that to do so is to play God. However, this charge is too broad, for it could encompass any medical intervention. For example, are surgeons playing God when they remove cancerous tumors to save lives or when physicians revive a person whose heart has stopped beating? This is not to say that sometimes the "playing God" charge might not be legitimate, but one needs to be careful about being too broad in making the charge.

> *Somatic-cell therapy is still*
> *in its experimental stage.*

One ethical consideration that can be raised concerning somatic-cell therapy is the fact that it is still in its experimental stage and therefore caution needs to be taken. The whole area of research ethics is outside of the scope of this chapter, but any research that employs experimentation on humans needs to follow careful guidelines. Some general guidelines are: (1) A Good Research Design — The experiment or research project must be well-designed to achieve its purpose and be scientifically sound. (2) The Balance of Harm and Benefit — An experiment should not be performed, or should be terminated

in midprogress, unless there is a good chance that benefits outweigh the harms to be inflicted. (3) Competence of the
Investigator — The researcher has adequate scientific training
and skill to accomplish the purposes of the research, along
with a high degree of professionalism necessary to care for the
subject. (4) Informed Consent — The patient has been given
the following information: (a) a fair explanation of the procedures to be followed and their purposes, including identification of any procedures that are experimental, (b) a description
of the attendant discomforts and risks reasonably to be
expected, (c) a description of the benefits reasonably to be
expected, (d) a disclosure of appropriate alternative procedures that might be advantageous for the subject, (e) an offer
to answer any inquiries concerning the procedures, and
(f) instruction that the person is free to withdraw his/her consent and to discontinue participation in the project or activity
at any time without prejudice to the subjects. (5) Equitable
Selection of Subjects — Fair distributive justice should be
maintained in all recruiting of research subjects. (6) Com-
pensation for Research-Related Injury — This seems to be the
least we can offer to those who voluntarily submitted to some
form of medical experimentation or research in order that all
mankind can benefit from the knowledge gained. Most
somatic-cell therapy is currently performed in laboratories
with institutional review boards to help guide the study in
accordance with these guidelines.

Germ-line therapy is a bit more controversial. More than
just the present patient will be affected by such therapy and
more needs to be considered. The obvious advantage of
germ-line therapy is its efficiency. As Leroy Walters says,
"Correcting a defect once, through germ-line therapy, and
having the correction passed on to the subject's descendants
might seem more reasonable than repeating somatic-cell gene
therapy generation after generation in a family afflicted by a
genetic disease."[36] However, the argument above concerning
experimental treatment has even more force in this situation.
One may not know for a number of generations if a particular germ-line treatment has been effective, or worse, if it is

causing other unforeseen damage. Therefore it is difficult to form an adequate design plan and to balance harms and benefits. The issue of informed consent is also raised by some, for we are now discussing performing experimental treatment on future generations who do not have any say in such experimentation.

Another problem with germ-line therapy is that it must be performed on embryos in order for the intervention to spread to all cells including reproductive cells. This causes two problems: first, much of the early work in laboratory animals has been unsuccessful, resulting in defective embryos and embryos that did not survive the therapy. It is highly probable that such therapy when used on humans will have a similar effect, at least in the beginning. Given the personhood of the fetus from conception, this means we would be creating defective children who would most likely be aborted, or simply killing the unborn. Second, some have suggested that germ-line therapy would work best if done in preimplantation screening. However, the same problem occurs here, for if the therapy is not successful during implantation the embryo will be discarded — aborted before even entering the womb. While I would not completely rule out the possibility of germ-line therapy, the present problems raise extreme difficulties that make such therapy on humans unjustifiable for the present.

The most controversial of the types of genetic intervention is any form of genetic enhancement, either somatic or germ-line. Many ethicists have argued that intervention to cure or prevent genetic disease may be acceptable, but any attempts to enhance one's capabilities on the genetic level would be ethically unacceptable. There are many reasons why people are against this. First, some argue that this really is playing God. God created man with certain abilities and limitations and to attempt to expand them is to step into a role that is reserved only for him. Second, this is utopian thinking — we are trying to create the perfect man and perfect society. Such utopian thinking does not take into account that man has a sin nature and will likely abuse such power if given the opportunity. The possibility of a world like *Gattaca* is very real. Third, it is too easy to shift from improving the individual to improving society. When we make such a shift, we have stepped completely out of the realm of the medical and into the political realm. This raises a fourth ethical issue, that of differing opinions of what is "enhancing." Who will decide this? Doctors, politicians, scientists, philosophers, theologians and lawyers may all feel qualified to make the decision.

All of the above problems are eclipsed by the main problem with enhancement, *eugenics*. Eugenics is the idea of improving the human race by gene selection and manipulation. There are two types of eugenics: negative and positive eugenics. Negative eugenics is the decreasing of undesirable or harmful genetic traits. Positive eugenics is the enhancing of genes to improve their functioning. While some are actually advocating eugenics, they will not usually use that term. The term "eugenics" has fallen on bad times. There is a reason for that.

Eugenics is the idea of improving the human race by gene selection and manipulation.

Usually when we think of eugenics we think of Nazi Germany during the days leading up to and including World War II. Actually the Nazi program can be traced all the way back to 1895 when Alfred Ploetz wrote a document on "racial hygiene." In it he attacked the "medical practice that helps the individual but endangers the race by allowing individuals, who would not have otherwise survived, to live and reproduce themselves."[37] At that time there was no knowledge of genetic intervention, so negative eugenics was performed by forced sterilization along with euthanasia. Positive eugenics was through breeding among the "elite." In 1933 Germany passed a mandatory sterilization law that was explicitly for eugenic purposes. Those sterilized were the mentally incompetent, severely retarded and the criminally insane — over 400,000 between 1934 and 1937.[38] In 1939 Hitler passed a law allowing for the euthanasia of members of the same group. Part of the purpose for such laws was economics. Germany was in the midst of a terrible depression and the government could not afford to pay for these persons in state-run facilities. However, the laws soon broadened to include others considered "socially undesirable" — the incurably ill, prostitutes, criminals, and certain races, including, as everyone knows, the Jews. It was only the end of the war that ended these practices.

Most of us are familiar with the Nazi record. What many Americans are not aware of is that eugenics was also being heavily promoted and accepted in Great Britain and in the United States. In fact the United States was at the forefront of the eugenics movement in the early part of this century. Margaret Sanger, founder of the birth control movement in this country, spoke throughout the world on behalf of eugenics. Her saying was, "More children for the fit, less for the unfit."[39] From 1907-1929, 28 states passed laws allowing the sterilization of those deemed mentally incompetent and criminally insane. This is years before Germany passed its laws. Over 15,000 individual Americans were sterilized, most against their will, while being incarcerated or in mental homes.

One of the most famous cases in American judicial history was the case of *Buck v. Bell*. The case was argued before the United States Supreme Court in 1927. Carrie Buck was a 17-year-old young woman living in Virginia, supposedly retarded (a matter of great dispute today), who had become pregnant outside of wedlock (she was actually raped by a member of the family who was taking care of her). After giving birth, it was decided that she was mentally incompetent and this had led to her "loose" lifestyle. Harry Laughlin, a well-known eugenics advocate, testified against Carrie saying that she belonged to the "shiftless, ignorant, worthless, class of anti-social whites of the South."[40] The case was appealed to the Supreme Court, who voted 8-1 to uphold the legality of the sterilization of Carrie Buck (who was sterilized about 2 miles from where I am sitting in Lynchburg, Virginia). In his opinion, Justice Oliver Wendell Holmes wrote the infamous line,

"Three generations of imbeciles is enough." He went on to state, "The principle that sustains compulsory vaccination is broad enough to cover cutting the fallopian tubes."[41] Attorney Paul Lombardo has written a convincing argument that the whole case of *Buck v. Bell* was fabricated from the beginning for the very purpose of bringing the eugenics issue before the Supreme Court and getting its blessing and approval.[42]

Toward the closing days of World War II, the world began to learn of the Nazi atrocities all in the name of "eugenics." The term began to disappear from the names of organizations, as it became associated with racism and Naziism. However, eugenics itself didn't end, and as genetic research began to grow in the '50s, '60s, and '70s, a new form of coercion began to appear arguing for genetic therapy and enhancement. Arthur Dyck writes:

> Currently, and in the future, eugenics in the United States is, and will be, voluntarily carried out by physicians and genetic counselors. Eugenics takes place in what are regarded as autonomous choices on the part of willing individuals. Without government interference, abuses and coercion occur and will continue to occur unless the ethical and legal climate changes markedly.[43]

What kind of coercion is Dyck talking about? The coercion comes from the geneticist's attitude itself. While condemning the Nazi eugenics on the one hand, geneticists are promoting genetic enhancement on the other hand. "Coercion need not come from governments, but from the very concepts that geneticists, physicians, and health professionals tend to share as they implicitly or explicitly practice negative eugenics."[44] Dyck demonstrates this by comparing the three primary principles behind Nazi eugenics with the 1978 book *On Human Nature* by E.O Wilson, a leading founder of sociobiology at Harvard University. All three principles can be found in Wilson's book. Dyck concludes, "The foregoing analysis leads me to one final set of observations. It is misleading to speak of the dangers of repeating the history of eugenics. Eugenics is not simply a matter of history. Eugenics is practiced today."[45]

It may not always be easy to tell where to draw the line between therapy and enhancement.

It is my conclusion that every effort should be made to avoid any kind of enhancement intervention. It may not always be easy to tell where to draw the line between therapy and enhancement, but I believe many cases are obvious. Some have tried to arrive at criteria. John Feinberg attempts to establish a theological criterion which states: "Any use of this technology to fight something in human beings that is clearly a result of the consequences of sin and living in a fallen world is morally acceptable."[46] James Peterson attempts to arrive at five criteria for distinguishing between therapy and enhancement: incremental progress, choice expanding, parent-directed, within societal boundaries, and by acceptable means.[47] While I believe the criteria set forth by both authors have problems, I believe they are a start in clarifying an important issue. In previous chapters we have said the goal of medicine is to cure, not to kill. In genetic intervention our aim should be to cure, not to enhance.

Genetic Research and Experimentation

Much of what we have already discussed can be placed under the category of "research and experimentation." However two final areas especially fit under this category. One is a research issue and the other an experimental issue.

The Human Genome Project

The research issue is the **Human Genome Project** (HGP). In the history of our country we have only had a small number of important national scientific projects that would rival the HGP. The Manhattan Project of the 1940s and the Apollo Space Project of the 1960s would be the closest comparisons. Inaugurated in January of 1990 as a joint project of the National Institute of Health and the Department of Energy, the HGP was estimated at the time to cost about 15 billion dollars and take about 15 years to complete.

As we said at the beginning of the chapter, in each cell are the 46 chromosomes containing the blueprints for the functioning of the entire human organism. Each of the 46 chromosomes contain about 100,000 genes and are made up of about 3–3.5 billion base pairs of DNA molecules. This whole structure taken together is called the *human genome*. The goal of the HGP is to map out the entire human genome. This will consist in identifying every gene and every base pair and determining the sequence in which they are ordered. Leroy Walters provides a good analogy to help understand the project:

> If you wanted to make a physical map of the Untied States, you might first use a satellite photograph to get an over view of the whole country. This satellite photo would correspond to locating the 23 pairs of chromosomes. Next you might divide the country into 1000 regions each comprising a certain number of square miles. For this more detailed map you might use photographs taken from airplanes. Similarly scientists will divide the human genome into major regions each of which will consist of 40,000 base pairs. In our geography project, there might be certain regions that require special attention even at this stage of mapping, for example, major metropolitan areas or areas with potentially dangerous geological faults. In a parallel way, scientists have already discovered that certain disease-related genes are located in particular regions of particular chromosomes. They will therefore subject these regions to special scrutiny at this stage of mapping. The final stage in the geography project might be a highly detailed map that indicates individual streets or even individual buildings on those streets. This fine level of detail would correspond to knowing the sequence in which some or all of the 3 to 3.5 billion base pairs are arranged in human chromosomes.[48]

One can imagine the length of time and how complicated such a detailed mapping of the United States would be, and streets and buildings can be easily seen and identified. Genes and DNA molecules don't have that advantage. The HGP is a massive project.

The first goal was to locate genetic "markers" which help localize specific genes. In 1990 it was estimated that they would need about 1500 markers and the goal was to find the markers by 1995. Francis Collins, a Christian geneticist working on the HGP, reports that this goal was completed in 1993 and they have found about 10,000 markers.[49] The second goal was to create a physical map of fragments of DNA that cover a particular region. The goal was to complete this stage by 1998. Collins reports that as of 1996, 96% of that goal was reached.[50] The third stage, sequencing the 3–3.5 billion base pairs of DNA, is the most ambitious phase of the HGP and will take the longest time. Collins reports that this part of the project was begun in earnest in 1996 and they expect to reach the goal by 2005, the projected year the HGP is to finish.[51]

With the HGP in full swing, new genes are being found on a regular basis and medical science is already benefitting from the project. For example, Collins reports that a gene for breast cancer was identified in 1994. They now know that a woman having this gene has a 50% risk of getting breast cancer by age 50, with a lifelong risk of 80%.[52] So far the main benefit of the HGP is diagnostic. It is helping to locate the genes that are involved in the 5,700 genetic disorders. This involves more than just single gene disorders. Many of these diseases involve complex relationships between different genes as well as environmental factors. At this time very little therapeutic value has come from the HGP, but the hope is that through gaining knowledge more means will be uncovered to do genetic intervention.

One aspect of the HGP program is ELSI — the Ethical, Legal and Social Implications division of the HGP. This division was specifically designed to consider the possible ethical and social implications of the HGP. The HGP itself actually introduces very few new ethical issues, but as new genes are discovered almost on a weekly basis, it does accelerate and compound many of the issues we have already discussed.

The biggest concern is information control and privacy. Once the human genome is mapped out, it will be possible for your entire DNA sequence to be known. Who will have access to this information? Insurance companies may decide they have a right, as may employers or the government. The opportunity for discrimination is highly possible and scenarios like those in *Gattaca* may happen.

> ## The biggest concern of HGP is information control and privacy.

The HGP also raises issues of commercialization due to genetic patenting. In 1980 the Supreme Court ruled in the case of *Diamond v. Chakrabarty*. The case involved a patent on a genetically altered strain of bacteria capable of breaking down crude oil. The United States Patent Office refused to give a patent to "living matter." The case came before the Supreme Court who determined that a genetically engineered microorganism was patentable. In 1987 an inventor attempted to patent a new type of oyster. At first he was denied, but on appeal he was granted a patent and the Patent office announced that nonnaturally occurring, nonhuman, multicellular organisms, including animals, were patentable. Within a year Harvard University was granted a patent on a mouse. By ten years after *Chakrabarty* over 7800 patent applications were on file for genetically engineered life forms.[53] In patenting a gene or genetic process, a biotech corporation would own the gene or process. The amount of income for biotech companies could be enormous. Sherry reports an estimated growth over the next 10 years of 40 billion dollars.[54] Many fear that knowledge gained through the HGP will fuel the fires of commercialization of genetic materials. So far the courts have not seemed to be willing to limit the expanding scope of patents. If limits are not placed on what private companies can patent, not only may therapeutic gene intervention become commercialized, but enhancement intervention may become a commercial reality for those willing to pay the price.

Finally, an area of concern of the HGP is eugenics. With information of the complete human genome the temptation to enhance individuals, as well as the human race, will be very difficult to fight. Jeremy Rifkin, a staunch opponent of genetic engineering, quotes a July 22, 1982, *New York Times* editorial as saying "that once scientists are able to repair gene defects 'it will become harder to argue against adding genes that confer desired qualities, like better health, looks or brains.' According to the *Times*, 'There is no discernible line to be drawn between making inheritable repairs of genetic defects and improving the species.'"[55]

Many think that such talk is irrational and that "we never would do that." One only need to be reminded of the shabby ethical record of research and experimentation in this country: the Tuskegee syphilis study, in which dozens of African-Americans were submitted to over 40 years of syphilis study by the government with no offer of therapeutic relief; the military studies on the effects of radiation poisoning by submitting hundreds of American military personnel to radiation exposure; the eugenics and involuntary sterilization program of the '20s and '30s that ended only because of its unpleasant association with Naziism. We need to be reminded of statements like the following by the Chief Justice of the United States, Oliver Wendell Holmes, in the *Buck v. Bell* case:

> We have seen more than once that the public welfare may call upon the best citizens for their lives. It would be strange if it could not call upon those who already sap the strength of the State for these lesser sacrifices often not felt to be such by those concerned, in order to prevent our being swamped with incompetence. It is better for all the world, if instead of waiting to execute degenerate offspring for crime or to let them starve for their imbecility, society can prevent those who are manifestly unfit from continuing their kind.[56]

And if one should think that *Buck v. Bell* was a long time ago and we have since learned our lesson, read this 1988 quote from Congress's Office of Technology Assessment on the ethcial and social implications of the HGP:

> Human mating that proceeds without the use of genetic data about the risks of transmitting diseases will produce greater mortality and medical costs than if carriers of potentially deleterious genes are alerted to their status and *encouraged to*

mate with non-carriers or to use artificial insemination or other reproductive strategies.[57]

None of this is to say that we should abandon the HGP. But it is saying that we may need to slow down and consider the abuses such information can lead to and to have a plan in place to confront those abuses before they might occur.

Cloning   On February 23, 1997, the world was stunned when an announcement was made that scientists of the Roslin Institute in Scotland, headed by embryologist Dr. Ian Wilson, had cloned a sheep which they named "Dolly." According to the institute, Dolly was the first successful clone of a mammal from a cell of an adult animal. She was derived from cells that had been taken from the udder of a 6-year-old Finn Dorsett ewe and cultured for several weeks in a laboratory. The researchers cultured 277 reconstructed eggs, each with a diploid nucleus, for 6 days in temporary recipients. Twenty-nine of the eggs that appeared to have developed normally to the blastocyst stage were implanted into surrogate Scottish Blackface ewes. Only one was born, Dolly, on July 5, 1996, about 148 days later.

> ### Scientists have been discussing the concept of cloning for decades.

The idea of cloning is not new, scientists have been discussing the concept for decades. Until recently, though, cloning was more the stuff of science fiction than of scientific fact. Because there has been such a wealth of fictional literature about cloning, most people's immediate reaction to Dolly was based on myth rather than facts. Some of these myths we should clear up right away. First, clones are not full-grown adults. They are embryos who have to go through the normal gestation period and grow and develop. Second, if there were human clones, they would have souls and be persons just like any other person conceived and born of human parentage. In fact, natural human clones already exist: identical twins. Each individual twin has the exact same genetic make up as the other twin. Yet each is an individual person with his or her own soul. Third, while a human clone would genetically be identical to its original, it wouldn't be the exact same person. There are a lot more things that go into forming your personality than your genetic makeup. Fourth, Dolly was not the first living thing ever cloned. Plants have been cloned, as have frogs. In 1993 there was even an attempt to clone a human embryo.

Exactly how does cloning work? There are a number of different kinds of cloning, some of which scientists have been doing for years. *Molecular cloning* occurs when scientists make clones of the DNA molecule for scientific study. This is a pillar of recombinant DNA and has led to the production of such medicines as insulin. *Cellular cloning* occurs when copies are made of cells and cultured in a laboratory. Since they are all of the same cell line, their genetic makeup is identical. Again this is a common laboratory procedure. The cloning procedure used to produce Dolly is a procedure known as **somatic-cell nuclear transfer**. First a cell is removed from a donor animal and placed in a bath of chemicals to keep it alive. Second, an unfertilized egg is removed from a female animal. Like all reproductive cells, the egg has a nucleus with half the chromosomes necessary for the egg to produce offspring. Third, scientists remove the nucleus from the egg. Fourth, they place the nucleus from the donor cell, which contains all the chromosomes from the donor, into the egg by "fusing" the egg and cell with an electronic jolt. This jolt also causes the egg to begin the process of dividing and reproducing. After a number days the embryo is then inserted into a female animal. The female gives birth to an exact genetic copy of the original donor. While this sounds simple, remember that they tried 277 times before they were able to come up with one sheep. There have been other successful animal clonings since Dolly, but failures are much more common than successes.

What are the benefits of cloning? First, there are a number of research benefits for cloning animals. Often scientists desire to test and research genetically identical animals, and cloning would help obtain such animals. Second, there is an obvious commercial importance in cloning animals. Cloning can increase reproductive output and the quality of livestock. The best animals can be cloned. Third, cloning would be very helpful in the production of "transgenic" livestock. This activity occurs when genes of one species are injected into a fertilized egg of a different species to produce tissues and other substances which can be of medical value, such as proteins and nutriceuticals (an improvement in the nutritional value of food, such as milk). Fourth, cloning could aid in the understanding of cell-differentiation and cell-based therapies. Fifth, an important use of cloning is that it could help in organ transplantation. If human organs can be cloned, then there would not be a shortage of organs. If the organ can be cloned from the person in need, then there wouldn't be the problem of rejection.

There are a number of research benefits for cloning animals.

When Dolly was first announced to the world, there was an immediate reaction. Spurred on by the media, people wondered, "If they could clone a sheep, are they far from cloning a human being?" Most response to the idea of cloning a human has been negative, though none of the scientists at the Roslin Institute even remotely suggested it. Within days of the announcement of Dolly, President Clinton issued a ban on federal funding related to any attempts to clone human beings. He also convened the National Bioethics Advisory Council and asked them for a report on the ethical implications of human cloning within ninety days. The NBAC interviewed scores of experts in the scientific, legal, bioethical and religious fields before submitting their report in June, 1997. The commission made the five following recommendations:

1. At this time it is morally unacceptable for anyone in the public or private sector, whether in research or clinical setting, to attempt to create a child using somatic-cell nuclear transfer.
2. Federal legislation [should] be enacted to prohibit anyone from attempting, whether in a research or clinical setting, to create a child through somatic-cell nuclear transfer cloning.
3. Any regulatory or legislative actions undertaken to effect the forgoing prohibition on creating a child by somatic-cell nuclear transfer should be carefully written so as not to interfere with other important areas of scientific research.
4. The federal government, and all interested and concerned parties, [should] encourage widespread and continuing deliberation on these issues in order to further our understanding of the ethical and social implications of this technology.
5. Federal departments and agencies concerned with science should cooperate in seeking out and supporting opportunities to provide information and education to the public in the area of genetics, and on other developments in the biomedical sciences, especially where these affect important cultural practices, values and beliefs.[58]

The NBAC's main reasons for calling for a federal ban on human cloning were: (1) it was not safe enough at this time and (2) time is needed to address serious ethical concerns. The federal ban applies only to federally funded institutions, however the NBAC requested that private institutions voluntarily comply with the recommendations.

While most are against human cloning, some have advocated it. Dr. Richard Seed, a geneticist in Chicago, announced in January 1998 that he would attempt to clone the first human being and would open a for-profit clinic for cloning humans. He claimed that, rather than being contrary to God's plan, cloning should be seen as a part of it: "God made man in His own image and His plan is that we should become one with God. . . . This is a significant step in the right direction."[59] Seed claimed that at the time he did not have the funds available to undertake the project but hoped some would step forward to fund his clinic. Most reaction to Seed was negative.

A number of ethical problems are raised with the possibility of human cloning. First, a number of ethicists have pointed out that right now any thought of cloning humans would be premature due to the safety factors. There are just too many unknowns still, and experimentation would result in a large number of dead or defective embryos. Recognizing that these are persons from the moment of conception means we would be submitting them to dangerous experimental treatment, killing many of them and causing defects that would either result in abortion or the birth of defective children. Such a scenario was made clear in a recent science fiction motion picture when a cloned person finds the laboratory in which she was cloned and sees all the previous versions of herself, hideously distorted, floating in tanks of chemicals. Cloning is presently too dangerous and, in fact, it is difficult to believe we will ever get to the level where we can be sure the first time we try cloning it will be successful. The benefits don't outweigh the harms.

A question exists as to what cloning will do to the individual psychologically.

Second, a question exists as to what cloning will do to the individual psychologically. Several ethicists have raised the issue of a loss of identity and uniqueness. Christian ethicist Gilbert Meilaender commented in his testimony before the NBAC:

> Our children begin with a kind of genetic independence of us, their parents. They replicate neither their father nor their mother. That is a reminder of the independence that we must eventually grant to them and for which it is our duty to prepare them. To lose even in principle this sense of the child as gift will not be good for children.[60]

Some have argued that there is no difference in "uniqueness" between a clone and a twin. However, Hans Jonas makes a case for the fact that there is a significant difference.[61] Contemporary twins begin their lives in "ignorance" of what will happen to the other or what choices the other will make. A clone does not have the same freedom. Jonas argues that the clone knows too much and the actions of his "original" are bound to have a psychological effect on him. The later twin will not have the spontaneity and authentic creativity the earlier twin had.

Third, many are concerned what effect cloning will have on the family unit. Social and legal questions arise concerning the clone's relation to the rest of the family. Who is the parent of the cloned child? Is it the parent of the original or is the original herself the parent? Is the original also the sibling of the clone? If a woman clones herself, does the child have a father? Some believe that ambiguity over parental roles may be harmful psychologically to a child's sense of identity. Others argue that this is not a severe problem as modern children are often dealing with complex relationships with divorce, assisted reproduction, same-sex relationships. However, this author has a hard time using the "modern" state of the family as the standard by which we should judge the ethics of cloning. The basic family unit of father and mother joined for life and raising children together in a loving and nurturing environment is biblically sound, historically justified and can be grounded in natural law. While it is true that tragic situations sometimes tear families apart, that should never be the standard by which we should judge new concepts.

Fourth, cloning can lead to the dangerous attitude of treating children as means to some end rather than ends themselves. There are a number of different levels to this problem. The NBAC recognizes the problem of cloning being an issue of illegitimate means of control over our offspring. There is the real concern that parents may be cloning children to meet certain expectations, like replacing a lost child, or to be a copy of themselves to accomplish the parents' goals, rather than the child's. The child ends up living for the sake of the parent instead of having a life of its own free from illegitimate parental constraints. On another level there is the fear that children will be cloned to provide organs or materials for other siblings in medical need. If an infant is in need of an organ, a child might be cloned, brought close to term, aborted, and have its organ removed and placed in the infant. Children become instruments to meet our needs rather than having value themselves.

> *Cloning can lead to the dangerous attitude of treating children as means to some end rather than ends themselves.*

Fifth, cloning could easily lead to discrimination as a new second class of citizens is created, the "cloned" ones. Greg Koukl comments: "Clones might be treated as less than human. The appropriate environment for a child is a family. Because of the unique origin of a child that is a clone, it will be tempting to claim she is truly a parentless child created by — and owned by — the scientist who simply assembled her biological parts. To treat a human being merely as property is deeply immoral."[62]

Finally, Leonard Kass suggests that we might not be able to articulate our specific reasons for what is wrong with cloning, but perhaps it is not always necessary to do so:

> Almost no one sees any compelling reason for human cloning. Almost everyone anticipates its possible misuses and abuses. Many feel oppressed by the sense that there is nothing to prevent it from happening and this makes the prospect seem all the more revolting. Revulsion is surely not an argument . . .But . . . in crucial cases repugnance is often the emotional bearer of deep wisdom beyond reason's power fully to articulate.[63]

Perhaps Gilbert Meilaender provides the best perspective for us as Christians. He appeared before the NBAC and delivered some remarks entitled "Begetting and Cloning." Meilaender spoke as a Christian theologian and remarked that:

> What Protestants found in the Bible was a normative view: namely that the sexual differentiation is ordered toward the creation of offspring, and children should be conceived from the marital union. By God's grace the child is a gift who springs from the giving and receiving of love. Marriage and parenthood are connected — held together in a basic form of humanity.[64]

Meilaender goes on to explain this Christian normative view by saying that procreation in the marriage sexual relationship is good for the relationship and it is good for the child. It is good for the sexual relationship because it is a reminder that sex has a purpose beyond just the personal pleasure of a couple. They are "procreating" (not "producing") and the sexual union states that there is something beyond just these two people at work here. Second, it is good for the child, for it is what unites the child to the parents in an eternal and sometimes mysterious bond. Meilaender appeals to the Nicene creed to explain this relationship:

> When Christians tried to tell the story of Jesus as they found it in their Scriptures, they were driven to some rather complex formulations. They wanted to say that Jesus was truly one with that God whom they call Father, lest it should seem that what he had accomplished did not really overcome the gulf that separates us from God. Thus while distinguishing the persons of Father and Son, they wanted to say that Jesus is truly God one being with the father. And the language in which they did this . . . is language which describes the Son of the Father as "begotten, not made." . . . What we beget is like ourselves, what we make is not, it is the product of our free decisions and its destiny is ours to determine. . . . If it is, in fact, human begetting that expresses our equal dignity, we should not lightly set it aside in a manner as decisive as cloning.[65]

In the end the question of human cloning comes down to dealing with who we are and who we want to be. I close with one final comment by Meilaender:

> We need the virtue of humility before the mystery of human personhood and the success of generations. We need the realization that the children who come after us are not simply a product for us to mold.[66]

For the sake of who we are, what we will be, and for our children, *Sola Deo Gloria.*

ENDNOTES

[1]This is a summary of the opening scenes of the 1997 motion picture *Gattaca*, written and directed by Andrew Niccol and produced by Danny DeVito, George Kacandes, Joshua Levinson, Michael Shamberg, and Stacy Sher. The title "Gattaca," which is the name of an aerospace firm in the picture, is composed entirely of the four letters that label the nucleotide bases in DNA — G,T,C,A.

[2]I am using a summary of Dawkins's analogy found in John Fletcher's *Coping with Genetic Disorders: A Guide for Clergy and Parents* (New York: Harper and Row, 1982), pp. 5-6. Dawkins's original analogy is in his book, *The Selfish Gene* (New York: Oxford University Press, 1976), pp. 23-24.

[3]Dawkins claims there is no architect, that this is all just chance and natural selection. However, if one considers his analogy to be precise, it seems to lead to the opposite conclusion. How many of us would argue that a real building, just like the one described here, could occur purely by chance? However, this is a topic for another book.

[4]Again, I am indebted to Fletcher's summary of this illustration, *Coping*, p. 11.

[5]I am indebted to my daughter Erin for this addition to the library illustration.

[6]Fletcher, *Coping*, pp. 11-14.

[7]Leroy Walters, "Reproductive Technologies and Genetics," in *Medical Ethics*, 2nd. ed., ed. by Robert M. Veatch (Boston: Jones and Bartlett, 1998), p. 220.

[8]Ibid.

[9]Walters, "Reproductive Technologies," p. 220. Walters makes a distinction between genetic testing and genetic screening, but for our purposes we will use them interchangeably.

[10]Ibid., p. 221.

[11]*In vitro* literally means "in glass" and refers to conceptions which occur outside of the mother's body in a science lab. These have erroneously been called "test tube" conceptions. They actually take place in a petri dish. After

conception, the zygote will be allowed to grow to the 4-8 cell stage and then be implanted in the mothers womb. Usually *in vitro* fertilizations are for those who need reproductive assistance. When performed, more than one egg is usually fertilized. Those not used are discarded.

[12]Gregory Pence, *Classic Cases in Medical Ethics*, 2nd ed. (New York: McGraw-Hill, 1995), p. 398.

[13]Ibid., p. 408.

[14]U.S. President's Commission for the Study of Ethical Problems in Medicine and Biomedical and Behavioral Research. "Screening and Counseling for Genetic Conditions" (Washington, DC: Government Printing Office, February 1983), p. 55.

[15]Scott Rae, "Prenatal Genetic Testing, Abortion, and Beyond," in *Genetic Ethics: Do the Ends Justify the Genes?* ed. by John F. Kilner, Rebecca D. Pentz, and Frank E. Young (Grand Rapids: Eerdmans, 1997), p. 138.

[16]Ibid., p. 140.

[17]Gilbert Meilaender, *Bioethics: A Primer for Christians* (Grand Rapids: Eerdmans, 1996), p. 49. Meilaender is quoting from Josef Pieper's book *About Love* (Chicago: Franciscan Herald Press, 1974), p. 19.

[18]Ibid.

[19]Rae, "Prenatal Genetic Testing," p. 141.

[20]Meilaender, *Bioethics*, pp. 55-56.

[21]Pence, *Classic Cases*, p. 402.

[22]C. Christopher Hook, MD, "Genetic Testing and Confidentiality," in *Genetic Ethics*, p. 127.

[23]Paul R. Billings, Mel A. Kohn, Margaret deCuevas, et. al., "Discrimination as a Consequence of Genetic Testing," *American Journal of Human Genetics*, 50:476-482 (1992).

[24]Hook, "Genetic Testing," p. 127.

[25]Ibid., p. 128.

[26]Carol Haas, "Genetic testing worms its way into firms' screening processes," *Atlanta Business Chronicle* (July 8, 1996).

[27]*Norman-Bloodsaw v. Lawrence*, U.S. 9th Circuit Court of Appeals, 96-16256.

[28]Walters, "Reproductive Technologies," p. 225.

[29]Dick Russell, "Genetic Engineering Is Dangerous," in *Genetic Engineering: Opposing Viewpoints*, ed. by William Dudley (San Diego: Greenhaven Press, 1990), p. 26.

[30]Nelson A. Wivel and LeRoy Walters, "Germ Line Gene Modification and Disease Prevention: Some Medical and Ethical Perspectives," *Science* 262: 533-536.

[31]Walters, "Reproductive Technologies," p. 229.

[32]Ibid.

[33]This quote by Willard Gaylin is on the screen at the beginning of the 1997 film *Gattaca*. I am unaware of the original source.

[34]Quoted in Ronald Munson, *Intervention and Reflection: Basic Issues in Medical Ethics* (Belmont, CA: Wadsworth Publishing, 1992), p. 419.

[35]Charles W. Colson, "Contemporary Christian Responsibility," in *Genetic Ethics*, p. 220.

[36]Walters, "Reproductive Technologies," p. 231.

[37]Arthur J. Dyck, "Eugenics in Historical and Ethical Perspective," in *Genetic Ethics*, p. 26.

[38]Ibid., p. 27.

[39]As quoted by Dyck, ibid., p. 26.

[40]Pence, *Classic Cases*, p. 389.

[41]*Buck v. Bell*, 274 U.S. 200 (1927).

[42]Paul Lombardo, "Three Generations, No Imbeciles: New Light on Buck v. Bell," NYU Law Review (April 1985): 30-62.

[43]Dyck, "Eugenics," p. 30.

[44]Ibid., p. 33.

[45]Ibid., p. 37.

[46]John Feinberg, "A Theological Basis for Genetic Intervention," in *Genetic Ethics*, p. 187.

[47]James C. Peterson, "Ethical Standards for Genetic Intervention," in *Genetic Ethics*, pp. 197-200.

[48]Walters, "Reproductive Technologies," p. 223.

[49]Francis Collins, "The Human Genome Project," in *Genetic Ethics*, p. 99.

[50]Ibid.

[51]Ibid.

[52]Ibid.

[53]Stephen F. Sherry, "The Incentive of Patents," in *Genetic Ethics*, p. 115.

[54]Ibid.

[55]As quoted by Feinberg, "Theological Basis," p. 184.

[56]*Buck v. Bell*, 274 U.S. 200 (1927).

[57]Quoted in George Annas, "Who's Afraid of the Human Genome?" *Hastings Center Report* (July/August 1989), p. 20, emphasis mine.

[58]*Cloning Human Beings*, Report and Recommendations of the National Bioethics Advisory Commission (Rockville, MD: Government Printing Office, June 1997), pp. iii-v.

[59]Richard Seed, Interview on the National Public Radio program, *All Things Considered*, January 6, 1998.

[60]Gilbert Meilaender, "Begetting and Cloning," *NBAC Report* (March 13, 1997).

[61]Hans Jonas, *Philosophical Essays: from Ancient Creed to Technological Man* (Englewood Cliffs, NJ: Prentice-Hall, 1974). Jonas's argument was presented to the NBAC.

[62]Greg Koukl, "Christians Are Getting Upset about Cloning for the Wrong Reasons," *Stand to Reason Newsletter* (May/June 1997).

[63]Leonard Kass, *NBAC Report*, p. 70.
[64]Meilaender, "Begetting."
[65]Ibid.
[66]Meilaender, *Bioethics*, p. 4.

References

Books and Sources on Genetic Ethics

Beauchamp, Tom L. and Leroy Walters. *Contemporary Issues in Bioethics*. 5th ed. Belmont, CA: Wadsworth Publishing, 1999. Chapter 8.

Dudley, William, ed. *Genetic Engineering: Opposing Viewpoints*. San Diego: Greenhaven Press, 1990.

Fletcher, John C. *Coping with Genetic Disorders: A Guide for Clergy and Parents*. San Francisco, CA: Harper and Row, 1982.

Hubbard, Ruth and Elijah Wald. *Exploding the Gene Myth*. Boston: Beacon Press, 1993.

Kilner, John F., Rebecca D. Pentz, and Frank E. Young. *Genetic Ethics: Do the Ends Justify the Genes?* Grand Rapids: Eerdmans, 1997.

Lammers, Stephen E. and Allen Verhey, eds. *On Moral Medicine: Theological Perspectives in Medical Ethics*. Grand Rapids: Eerdmans, 1987. Chapter 12.

Mappes, Thomas A. and David Degrazia, eds. *Biomedical Ethics*. 4th ed. New York: McGraw-Hill, 1996. Chapter 91.

McGee, Glenn, ed. *The Human Cloning Debate*. (Berkeley, CA: Berkeley Hills Books, 1998).

——————. *The Perfect Baby: A Pragmatic Approach*. Lanham, MD: Rowman and Littlefield, 1997.

Meilaender, Gilbert. *Bioethics: A Primer for Christians*. Grand Rapids: Eerdmans, 1996.

Munson, Ronald. *Intervention and Reflection: Basic Issues in Medical Ethics*. Belmont, CA: Wadsworth Publishing, 1992. Chapter 7.

National Bioethics Advisory Council. *On Cloning Human Beings*. Rockville, MD: Government Printing Office, 1997.

Pence, Gregory E. *Classic Cases in Medical Ethics*. 2nd ed. New York: McGraw-Hill, 1995. Chapter 16.

——————. *Classic Works in Medical Ethics: Core Philosophical Readings*. New York: McGraw-Hill, 1998. Chapter 10.

Rae, Scott. B. *Brave New Families: Biblical Ethics and Reproductive Technologies*. Grand Rapids: Baker, 1997.

Ramsey, Paul. *The Fabricated Man: The Ethics of Genetic Control*. New Haven, CT: Yale University Press, 1970.

Robertson, John A. *Children of Choice: Freedom and the New Reproductive Technologies*. Princeton, NJ: Princeton University Press, 1994.

Veatch, Robert. *Medical Ethics*. 2nd ed. Sudbury, MA: Jones and Bartlett, 1907. Chapter 8.

Websites on issues in Genetic Ethics

"**Are Genetics Going Too Far?**"(http://www.op.net/~consys/SciWeb/Main. htm) — Interesting series of short articles by Lavinia.

"**Begetting and Cloning**" (http://www.firstthings.com/ftissues/ft9706/ meilaender.html) Gilbert Meilaender's excellent remarks to the National Bioethics Advisory Committee on human cloning.

"**Brave New World of Cloning**"(http://www.ucalgary.ca/UofC/eduweb/virtualembryo/cloning.html) — a fairly scientific article that may be difficult, but is very good. Includes links to other cloning resources.

"**Cloning and Ethics**"(http://www.interlog.com/~syedma/clone_ethics0.html) — another article on cloning.

Ethics Updates: Reproductive Technologies and Genetics (http://ethics. acusd.edu/reproductive_technologies.html) — another great site from Lawrence Hinman with links, resources and full text online articles.

Genetics and Ethics Home Page (http://www.ethics.ubc.ca/brynw/) — This page is run by a graduate student and can be fairly academic, but has good information.

"**Human Cloning — Supermodels, Sheep & Genes**" (http://people.delphi. com/patrickdixon/clonech.htm) — Good article on human cloning by Dr. Patrick Dixon. Watch out for all the ads for his book.

National Bioethics Advisory Committee (http://bioethics.gov/cgi-bin/ bioeth_counter.pl) — This is the home page for the NBAC, and you can read the report on human cloning here as well as other bioethics issues.

Primer on Molecular Genetics (Department of Energy) (http://www.ornl.gov/ TechResources/Human_Genome/publicat/primer/intro.html) — This is a great resource for learning the basics of genetics and genetic diseases.

"**Should We Clone Humans?**" (http://www.op.net/~consys/SciWeb/ ShouldWe.htm) — Another article on cloning, author unknown.

GLOSSARY

absolutism — the ethical view that some moral rules are always binding and universally apply to all people at all times in relevant circumstances.

act utilitarianism — a type of utilitarianism that is concerned only with fulfilling the greatest happiness for the greatest number within a particular situation; it does not appeal to any rules or general guidelines to determine the right act, but only to the consequences in that specific situation.

active euthanasia — the intentional and direct killing of another human life either out of motives of mercy, beneficence, or respect for personal autonomy; sometimes called mercy killing. In active euthanasia it is the action of the agent that is the direct cause of death in the subject.

advanced directive — a set of instructions from a competent, autonomous, informed person regarding decisions about future medical treatment in the event that the person becomes incapable of making a decision at a future time.

altruism — unselfish regard for the welfare of others; other-regarding actions.

anencephaly — a failure of the neural tissue to completely close at the *cephalic* or top end of the neural system; the cerebral cortex or upper level of the brain is missing but the brain stem is always present.

autonomy — derived from the Greek "autos" (self) and "nomos" (rule, governance, law); personal rule of the self while remaining relatively free from both controlling interferences by

289

others and personal limitations, such as inadequate understanding, that prevent meaningful choice.

baby doe laws — a group of 1983 federal regulations based on Section 504 of the Rehabilitation Act of 1973 mandating that all hospitals which practiced infanticide would lose all federal funding.

basic inherent capacity — the capacity that all humans have to function as persons by nature of their being human beings; the basic inherent capacity is present from the moment of conception though it may be in latent form due to undevelopment or a damaged/defective neurological system.

beneficence — the moral obligation to act for the benefit of others; more specifically, it is to act in a manner to further the legitimate interests of others.

best interest standard — a standard employed for making a decision for an incompetent patient where the decision is made by a proxy in light of what is deemed in the best interests of the patient according to an accepted general standard. This would include areas such as relief of suffering and preservation of life.

bioethics — the analysis and study of ethical issues and problems which arise due to the interrelationship between the practice of the medical/biological sciences and the rights and values of human beings.

casuistry — a method of doing bioethics that believes moral reasoning must begin from particular concrete situations; casuistry begins with a pardigmatic case and, rather than appealing to moral rules or principles, identifies relevant salient features in that case that are analogous to other cases.

categorical imperative — principle formulated by Immanuel Kant for determining the right thing to do in a given situation; one formulation is, "Act according to that maxim by which you can, at the same time, will that it should be a universal law."

cloning — the act of reproducing an exact genetic duplicate of a living thing.

consequentialism — any ethical theory in which the primary emphasis in determining if an act is right or wrong is the consequences or results of the action.

cultural determinism — the concept that our ideas about morality are completely dependent on the culture in which we have been raised.

death — the cessation of the essential characteristics and capacities that are necessary and sufficient conditions in order for a person to be alive.

decisive moment theory — theory concerning the personhood of the unborn which claims that there is a decisive moment in the pregnancy when the person comes into existence; there are eight possible decisive moments pointed to as possible events when the person could come into existence.

deontology — any ethical theory that looks at our actions and declares them right or wrong in themselves regardless of consequences; the primary emphasis is placed on the actions themselves.

divine command theory — ethical theory that proposes that our ethical duties are grounded in the commands of God. Since commands are always verbal, this means that one has to have some form of verbal divine revelation to inform one of God's commands. This revelation is the authoritative basis for all ethical duties.

DNR — "do not resuscitate"; a medical order placed in the patient's chart stating that, in the event of a cardiac or pulmonary arrest, resuscitative measures such as CPR, intubation and pharmaceutical interventions not be employed; DNR orders are a standard procedure in hospitals when it is determined that resuscitative efforts would be futile and only prolong the dying process; DNR decisions should always be made as an agreement between physicians and patients or patient surrogates.

durable power of attorney — a person, designated in advance by the patient, to act as a proxy decision-maker at the time that the patient is no longer able to make decisions concerning his own welfare.

ecogenetics — newer area of genetic research which studies situations in which it is not just a single gene that causes a genetic disorder but a combination of the genetic and environmental agents that are encountered.

egoism — a consequentialistic ethical theory which is concerned primarily about the ultimate consequences for self;

there are two types of egoistic theories, psychological egoism and ethical egoism.

essentialism — the view which says that morality is based on the nature of God; morality is derived from his very essence; as opposed to voluntarism.

ethic of care — a method of bioethics that began primarily in feminist writings and emphasizes responsibilities within relationships as the primary methodology in discovering what our moral actions should be; care ethics is relationship-based as opposed to principle-based or case-based.

ethical theory — an organized and coherent system of normative rules usually flowing out of, or traceable back to, one overall unifying axiom.

ethical egoism — an ethical theory which claims that we ought to act in a manner that ultimately serves our best interest; ethical egoism recognizes that it is possible to do an altruistic act, but one never should; as opposed to psychological egoism.

eugenics — the idea of improving the human race by gene selection and manipulation; negative eugenics is the decreasing of undesirable or harmful genetic traits while positive eugenics is the enhancing of genes to improve their functioning.

euthanasia — literally "good death"; any act of relieving a person of the burdens of excessive medical treatment which one knows, with a high degree of reasonable probability, will result in the person's death; two types: active and passive.

extraordinary means — a term often used to describe those medicines, treatments, and procedures that are not ordinary because they involve excessive burdens on the patient and do not offer reasonable hope of benefit.

fallibilism — concerning morality, a recognition of the possibility that our own view of morality could be wrong and other views of morality could be right.

force majeure — French for "superior force"; a legal term for an event or effect that cannot be reasonably anticipated or controlled.

functionalism — view of human personhood that defines person as one who presently functions, or can immediately function, according to a certain set of criteria.

genetic intervention — medical intervention on the genetic level by manipulating, inserting or replacing genetic material for therapeutic or enhancement purposes.

genetic screening — the use of diagnostic procedures for determination of the presence or absence of one or more genetic traits or conditions in an individual.

germ cells — the cells that become sperm and egg which contain the genetic information that will be passed on to future generations.

germ-line therapy — an intervention in the reproductive cells to attempt to modify them so that a particular genetic disorder would not be passed on to future generations.

gradualism — the view that says there is no one specific moment when personhood begins; personhood develops gradually over the entire pregnancy; in the beginning, at conception, there is no person and by the end, at birth, there is a person.

harm — the obstruction or prevention of the legitimate interests of one party by the invasive actions of another party.

hippocratic oath — oath attributed to Hippocrates (5th century BC) which has been considered foundational for medical ethics and is still often recited by graduating medical students.

human genome project — a government funded program whose goal is to map out the entire human genome; the project consists in identifying every gene and every base pair and determining the sequence in which they are ordered.

hurt — an awareness of either physical, emotional or psychological pain.

in vitro **fertilization** — literally, "in glass"; the process of fertilizing an egg with a sperm outside of the uterus in a petri dish and then placing the product in a uterus to develop naturally.

incommensurable — two or more things that cannot be compared because there is no common measure or standard of comparison between them.

infanticide — the intentional taking of a newborn's life; often out of mercy, but historically for a number of reasons such as physical abnormalities, sex selection, economic considerations, and social considerations.

inference — the relationship between the premises and conclusion of an argument; when an inference is present, it is said that the premises "lead to" the conclusion, or that the conclusion "follows from" the premises.

intention — the willful aim of a particular action.

justification — the process of appealing to reasons or premises as support for beliefs that one holds or judgments one makes.

justice — the maintenance of what is just by the impartial judgment of conflicting claims and the assignment of merited rewards or punishments.

kantian deontology — deontological ethical theory based on the teachings of Immanuel Kant who held that the only proper motive for action is the good will and that the morally right action could be determined by the categorical imperative.

latent capacity — a capacity that is present but, due to undevelopment or a damaged/defective neurological system, is not presently able to function.

living will — a document that expresses an individual's preferences for treatment to be in force should the person become incompetent and not be able to express their desires for end-of-life care.

meiosis — a process that takes place in the reproductive cells in which pieces of each chromosome inherited from an individual's father change places with matching chromosomes from his mother.

metaethics — the study of the meaning of ethical terms, moral justification, and the nature of value judgments.

minimalistic ethic — an ethical view that holds to only one norm, usually the harm of others, and is open to all other actions and values apart from that norm.

moral relativism — the ethical view that there are no objective or universal moral standards; morality is either individually or culturally determined.

motive — the attitude one has toward an action.

natural law theory — an ethical theory that holds that all men have a built-in capacity in their human nature to distinguish right and wrong; the basic idea of natural law is that everything that exists has a nature and the purpose of all things is to function in accordance with that nature.

nature — also essence; that which makes something to be the kind of thing it is as in human nature or divine nature.

negative rights — also called a "right of noninterference"; it is a right to make autonomous choices and to act on them without interference from others; also called liberty rights; the majority of our constitutional rights are negative rights.

neocortical death — a view of death where a person is determined as dead when the outer layer of the brain covering the cerebrum, the neocortex, has irreversibly ceased to function.

neonaticide — the killing or allowing of a severely impaired infant to die while under medical care; medical infanticide.

nontherapeutic abortion — abortion for any reason other than the health of the mother.

nonmaleficence — the obligation to avoid harming or injuring others.

normative ethics — a type of reasoning which makes moral judgments by appeals to norms, rules or principles.

ordinary means — term used to describe all medicines, treatments, and procedures that offer a reasonable hope of benefit without placing undue burdens on a patient (pain or other serious inconvenience).

passive euthanasia — the withholding or withdrawing of a life-sustaining treatment when certain justifiable conditions obtain and the patient is allowed to die from the debilitation or disease.

persistent vegetative state — a condition of permanent unconsciousness in which the person is completely unaware of himself or his surroundings though he may appear to be awake and go through regular sleep/wake cycles; it is usually the result of permanent neocortical impairment and is considered irreversible.

person — a living being that has the essential capacity for rational thought, emotional expression, willful direction, and moral reflection concerning him/herself and the world around him/her.

physician-assisted suicide — the intentional assistance of a physician in helping a patient to end his life through the provision of information and/or means necessary for them to accomplish that goal.

pluralistic relativism — the recognition that there are in fact many different cultures each with their own separate ethical and social values and, therefore, all views must be accepted as having an equal claim to being "right."

positive rights — rights that impose a positive duty on someone; a right that a person has to have something provided to him or her; as opposed to a negative right, others must actively provide something to him or her.

preemptive suicide — suicide which is undertaken not out of current suffering, but in anticipation of a predictably long, drawn-out decline in an illness.

premise — the reasons in an argument or in a justification.

prima facie — literally "at face value"; a right or duty which holds in normal cases unless it conflicts with a stronger or more fundamental right or duty, in which case the normal right or duty can be overridden by that which is stronger or more fundamental.

principle of double effect — a principle of morality which states that one action can have two effects — one good and one evil and as long as the good effect was the intended effect, the evil effect does not count against one.

principlism — a method of bioethics that begins with established principles or rules and then applies them to a particular ethical situation.

proportianalism — the view that every action is a mixture of good and evil, and therefore one should choose actions in which there is a greater balance of good over evil.

psychological egoism — ethical theory that holds that all our actions are ultimately done out of our own self-interest; psychological egoism claims that we have no choice, we have to act ultimately for self.

reflective equilibrium — as is used in this book, a process of balancing new information or insights a moral event may present, one's immediate moral judgments, and the three different aspects of a properly prioritized pluralistic ethical theory with the goal of maintaining a proper balance or state of equilibrium in one's moral life. (The term originated with John Rawls whose meaning is somewhat different from that used in this book.)

respect for autonomy — recognizing that persons have the freedom to make choices concerning decisions and treating them in such a way as to allow them to freely make their choices.

right — a justified claim that individuals or groups can make upon others or upon society.

rule utilitarianism — a type of utilitarianism which holds that general rules can be formed that usually provide the greatest happiness for the greatest number of people and that these rules can guide one in each situation he encounters.

sentience — the ability to feel physical pain.

somatic-cell nuclear transfer — a cloning process by which a cell is removed from a donor animal, the nucleus is removed from it, and the nucleus is then placed in an unfertilized egg of a female animal which has had its nucleus removed.

somatic cells — all the cells in the human body that contain genetic information not passed on in reproduction; as opposed to germ cells.

substituted judgment standard — a standard employed for making a decision for an incompetent patient where the decision is made by a proxy who attempts to be a substitute for the patient himself in light of the patient's specific wishes and desires; as opposed to the best interest standard, the patient's own values are allowed to shape the decision.

suicide — the intentional taking or forfeiting of one's life primarily for self-serving motives.

surcease suicide — suicide which is done as an escape from current suffering; as opposed to preemptive suicide.

teleological view of creation — the view that creation has been designed to function in a certain manner.

therapeutic abortion — an abortion performed to protect the health or life of the mother.

utilitarianism — the ethical theory that says the morally right thing to do is that which provides the greatest happiness to the greatest number of people.

viability — the time when a baby can begin to live outside of the special environment of the uterus, currently 20-22 weeks gestation.

virtue ethics — the ethical theory that morality should be conceived as primarily concerned not with acts or consequences, but with the cultivation of moral virtues or traits of character.

virtue — an "excellence"; in a moral sense, a trained behavioral disposition to continually live in a good and righteous manner, a manner of moral excellence.

voluntarism — the view that morality is based on the will of God; what makes something good is that God simply wills it so.

whole brain death — the absence and complete irrecoverability of all spontaneous brain activity and all spontaneous respiratory functions.